Words of praise
CANCER AND FAITH...

"This book is a journal of seeking and believing; it is as honest and realistic as it is prayerful. It will serve as a challenging and comforting companion, not only for the terminally ill and those who accompany them, but for all of us who are wayfarers in hope."

Rev. John Heagle, Co-Director
Therapy and Renewal Associates
Seattle, Washington

"When you buy this book, save yourself time and buy several copies because after reading the first page you will think of friends and family members (ill and well) who will be grateful for this astonishing gift of raw honesty in the face of human limitation.

"John Carmody finds words reserved for only a few human beings about experiences we all know but cannot talk about because we often do not know how. The act of reading this book is itself a healing, and as a literary effort, this book is destined to live forever."

Doris Donnelly
Author, *Spiritual Fitness*
Winner of 1994 Christopher Book Award

"No matter how one views death, it is always an interruption, an event arousing conflicting emotions in each of us. John Carmody makes you stare at death without blinking. 'Death,' he says, 'could be Christ's welcoming kiss.'"

Tim Unsworth
Author and columnist
Chicago, Illinois

"This book is a great gift to us from a gifted writer. From a body filled with cancer, John Carmody lets God know what it is like to live with excruciating pain, with fear, with concern for his beloved wife. He unabashedly tells God of his passionate love, and asks to see God's own loving care even in his suffering and illness. There is much here for reflection and prayer."

William A. Barry, S.J.
Provincial, Society of Jesus
New England Province

"*Cancer and Faith* is about the deepening of John Carmody's friendship with God. It is not about illness as such, but about illness as the occasion of an enhanced spirituality. The results are always faith-filled, sometimes romantic, occasionally sentimental, usually earthy and humorous."

Lisa Sowle Cahill
Professor of Theology
Boston College

"This is the real thing. A writer, timeless as the psalmist, enables us to walk through the valley of the shadow without blinking, but without fear as well."

Eugene Kennedy
Professor of Psychology
Loyola University, Chicago

"John Carmody does not so much speak about cancer as allow us to live through his cancer with all its pain and struggle. There are no pious platitudes, but there is an honest search for God where life seems to fall apart. I am grateful for John's invitation to journey with him in the pages of this book toward the God in whom we live and in whom we die."

Cornelius J. van der Poel, C.S.Sp.
Director, Health Care Ministry Program
Barry University, Miami Shores, Florida

"This book will be a source of wisdom to all who read it, but particularly to those who experience their own limits of life and death."

Margaret A. Farley
Professor of Christian Ethics
Yale University

"If creativity is a matter of shedding new light on old problems, John Carmody has written a masterfully creative book. This book brought tears to the eyes of his old teacher. Thank you, John Carmody, for making us more sober about death without being somber."

Jack McCall, S.J.
Clinical Psychologist
University of North Carolina

CANCER
AND
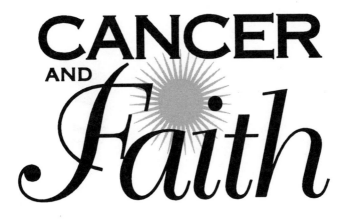
Faith

JOHN CARMODY

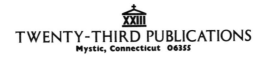
TWENTY-THIRD PUBLICATIONS
Mystic, Connecticut 06355

Twenty-Third Publications
185 Willow Street
P.O. Box 180
Mystic, CT 06355
(203) 536-2611
800-321-0411

ISBN 0-89622-594-1
Library of Congress Catalog Card Number 94-60080
Printed in the U.S.A.

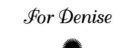

For Denise

Preface

Cancer is the aberrant growth of cells. It is often lethal, and most people find the word frightening. I was diagnosed as having multiple myeloma, a cancer of the bone marrow, in mid-April of 1992. Presently, multiple myeloma is not curable. The mean time of survival, from diagnosis to death, is about three years.

This book collects reflections and impressions about the interaction between my cancer and my Christian faith. The first group of reflections (1-24) come from 1992, shortly after my diagnosis. The second group (25-49) come from more than a year later, when I was finishing a first course of chemotherapy that had reduced the quantity of multiple myeloma enough to qualify as a partial remission. The two groups of reflections exhibit different psychologies. The first reflects the shock of a person newly informed that he is very ill. The second reflects a year's worth of living with a terminal illness, making its thorough acquaintance.

Susan Sontag has dealt well with the matter of serious illness and the metaphors that we attach to it. In recent

American history "cancer" has been more than a malignant biological process, because of the symbolisms we have hung over it. We did the same with tuberculosis a century ago and lately we have been dealing with AIDS in a similar way.

How we think about serious phenomena is as essential to their meaning as what they are physically in themselves. Meaning is cultural as much as it is natural or physical. Somehow, "cancer" seems to evoke more fright than "heart disease," though often the latter can threaten our lives more immediately. The idea that something in us is growing against us makes us seem a house divided, a body bent on self-destruction. Dealing with cancer well requires handling these metaphoric overtones. Treating the mind can be as important to the patient's well-being as administering chemotherapy. In presenting some reflections on cancer prompted by my Christian faith, I hope to treat the minds of some fellow believers to invitations to hope.

I have hated having cancer, but my faith has chanted that my hatred ought to stay measured. If God has determined that myeloma should shape my last years, who am I to kick against such a goad? If I cannot find blessings in this disposition of God, occasions for insight and purification, my faith is unimpressive.

God rules all our times, all our fates. The Father of Jesus makes his sun to shine, his rain to fall, on just and unjust alike. Not a hair of our heads falls without his awareness of it. All his works are works of love. These are elementary principles in the faith professed by Jesus. They supported him when he felt most abandoned and led him to the resurrection. These same beliefs are prominent in this book, and I invite all readers to entertain them. Indeed, I invite all readers to test them. Try them, as samples of God's providence. Turn them over, in good times and bad, and see whether they lighten your own mortality. I pray that they will.

Contents

Part Two

Part One

1. It Cannot Be Cured...

"The CAT scan confirms my fears. You have bone cancer. It cannot be cured." The voice was the voice of my doctor, but the words were yours, my God.

In ultimate matters, death and life, there are no intermediate causes. If we believe that you made the world and that you give being to each creature, we live or die at your behest. While philosophers and theologians can debate this proposition, it is beyond dispute for people of faith.

Unless we can abandon ourselves to your providence, O God, and believe that you number every hair of our heads, we cannot hold the faith given us by the Christian saints, cannot pass along the sacred treasure. Indeed, we must abandon the name of Jesus, who commended his spirit, his whole self, into your hands, sure that when asked for bread you would not give him a stone, when needing an egg he would not receive a serpent.

So I accuse you, God, only you, of this death sentence, and I bless you for it. All your ways are ways of love. My cancer must be a gift, a special token of your care. I weep to think it could be. Tears run down my cheeks. Is it possible you could not wait to have me with you in heaven, but had to speed things up? Let me not be foolish, God, but let me also cling to this consolation. I need it terribly.

My life has been sinful, imperfect, nothing I'm ready to let you judge. If you are not the father of prodigal children, the mother who can never abandon the child she has nursed, I have no hope. Give me hope, my God. Let my tears not flow in vain.

2. Sister Death

The mental image of Sister Death looms large in my mind as I confront my mortality and imminent death. Saint Francis of Assisi saw Sister Death, like Brother Sun and Sister Moon, as one of your creatures, O God, ministering your love to us.

The image of Sister Death does not completely satisfy me, however. I take greater comfort in the eucharist. By eating Christ's flesh and drinking his blood I do not so much turn his substance into my own as find myself taken over by his divine life. The trinitarian light and love dwell in the depths of my soul, glow at the *scintilla animae*.

I need my death to be your unmediated action, O God. I need to think of this terminal illness as your touch, your increasingly intimate embrace, your deliberately chosen way of freeing me from bodily limitations so that I might become lost and found in your infinity.

You are our truest being, even our truest selfhood. Our time is but a flash. Your eternity, making possible our time, is endless all at once. What you are we are, fractionally. At death we become what you are less fractionally, more completely. Come God, my death. Kill in me all that resists you, who are love. Teach me finally to love my life, my body, my world, now that they are ending. Help me to place them all in your keeping.

I want to abandon myself, as all lovers do, even though I am afraid. I cannot do it myself. You must continue to do it for me, in me, as you have been. O God, you are not too strange to be believed but too good. Who could think you love us, scruffy shabby sinful us, and make us divine? Who has been your counselor, God?

3. Three Levels of Reality

William Johnston's *Letters to Contemplatives* reminds me that human reality has at least three distinct levels. Physical reality is the world of nature and our bodies. Psychic reality is the world of images, thoughts, and feelings that we create by interacting with physical reality as agents who are more than physical. Spiritual reality is our deepest zone, level, or characteristic — the substantial self that is more than our thoughts and feelings. Spiritual reality is the whole of our being as held by you, our God, as hinged into you.

Much of the action and passion trafficking in spiritual reality goes forward in darkness and unknowing, in silences and darts of affection. This is the traffic that has always fascinated me. This is where I want to focus my preparation for you, my death. Without neglecting the physical and psychic levels of healing, I want to focus on the spirituality of terminal illness and preparation for death.

At the physical level, I feel obliged to undergo medical procedures like radiation and chemotherapy, if those specializing in bodily health recommend them. I want to be a cooperative patient, if only to honor your gift of life, my God.

Excellent books by Bernie Siegel, Norman Cousins, and other respected authors deal with the interplay of mind and body, or with emotional health in time of sickness. They seem to help many readers.

My consolation, however, comes from contemplating you, my God, and applying my senses to Christ on the cross. There you reknit my bones, even as they fray toward pathological fracture. There you heal the pains most worrying me: my sins of lust, sloth, ingratitude — most of all ingratitude.

You have heaped good things upon me. Above all you have given me Christian faith. Yet I have been careless, casual, inadvertent. You have been passionately naked, wholly vulnerable and available, and I have preferred pleasure, success, distraction.

Christ died for me. Each day he nourishes me with his body and blood. Yet I forget, don't pay attention, refuse to stir from my torpor. If nothing else, God, now you have gotten my attention. I am still far from properly grateful or attentive, but I have finally realized that time is short and my distance from you is long.

Let each pain be a reminder. Let each pill and medical procedure teach me again to nourish my hope that you are invading my body and interrupting my peaceful existence for a reason. Let my dying not be in vain.

4. My Spouse Suffers, Too

My dying is not mine alone. Already you have made that plain to me, O God. It changes my wife's life as much as mine. It shadows all her waking moments.

How tenderly she treats me. Who would have thought she would have to dress me, run all the errands, learn all the tricks of money and financial planning. Suddenly, she finds herself on a new track, in a new territory, without a map. We must rework all our old arrangements.

It helps that we never lived for the future, never planned a different life for retirement. But we also never planned for separation. If your coming in death separates my spirit from my flesh, what does it do to the other half of my soul, the woman with whom I've become one flesh?

I find it interesting that my sins against my spouse are like my sins against you, my God. I have not appreciated her as I ought. Often I have taken her for granted, not seen the wonder of her love.

Her character does not predominate among contemporary women. She is old fashioned, made for one man. Now she is like a mother bear protecting her cub. When she weeps in desolation, I feel guilty of abandonment.

We're striving mightily to treasure our last days together. We're also reconsidering the traditional images of heaven, like the one given in Chapter 22 of Matthew's Gospel. In heaven there has to be giving and taking in marriage just as there have to be rich friendships. Otherwise, the resurrection of Jesus does not bring all of creation into your heavenly household. We need to hope that we shall find complete fulfillment in your heaven, in your divine life all the good things of your creation.

Heaven has to be the consummation of everything you have given us on earth. The new Jerusalem must be the old Jerusalem perfected. It must be all that the best prayers in the Temple, the best embraces of the lovers in the *Song of Songs*, sought and adumbrated.

Marriage is a profound manifestation of your love for us, not something you can discard as you transform us from our earthly existence to heaven. When I kiss away her tears, I have to know my wife will be with me always. How else can I repay her for so much love?

5. It's Good to Cry

The friend whose call most moved me is the one who sobbed full out, brokenheartedly. Our note telling of my illness drew from him a revelation of love we could not have imagined. Many of the women who called were teary, but this man exposed his grief nakedly. Because he did, we could console him.

As I've found again and again, my God, you treasure our vulnerability. You do not baby us, but you stand against our self-sufficiencies. Women seem to know this better than men. But now you are teaching me, even giving me a measure of the gift of tears. An Eastern Orthodox spiritual father once said that no one ought to be able to approach the eucharist without weeping. He did not mean in sorrow only. He was not stressing lamentation for sins. He had in mind tears of joy, being overwhelmed by your goodness.

Your beauty, my God, has often moved me to tears. Let fine liturgical music play five minutes and my eyes are sure to glisten. Now I cry for the poignancy of creation, the vulnerability of all life.

When this sickness arrived, I thought of my father, wasted by prostate cancer twenty years ago. He died with a beatific smile early one New Year's Day, like an El Greco saint gracing a new calendar. Kneeling at his coffin, I thought of all his sufferings, and the tears gushed out of me. Now he was finally at rest, in peace, having died well, with courage, dignity, and great faith. I wondered whether his dying hadn't been a final gift to me. He seemed to be saying, "Fear not. Death can be your friend." Since then I've not feared death deeply nor been uncomfortable around the dying.

It's disturbing to realize that I love the intensity death brings, the ruthless excision of nonessentials. Keep me, good God, from foolish confidence, the wrong kind of zest. Keep me humble, well aware that I am no hero when it comes to pain, fully conscious that I have no holiness to defend me from your refining fire. Look not on my sins, but on the faith of your church. Even though my institutional membership is hedged, I want to be part of your communion, another link in your great chain of tradition and witness. I want to die as one of your people, a son who did not despise the mother who gave him faith even though he subordinated her to you more than many of her leaders thought good.

6. My Body Crumbles

It feels strange to be immobile. Once I ran down the stairs, swam hundreds of laps, loved long leisurely walks. Now I limp on swollen feet, painful legs, inching ahead with a four-pronged cane. In a month you have taken away my motion, my quickness. My mind still squirts forward. My tongue is ready enough. But my body drags. The whole lower half of me is heavy, nearly dysfunctional.

Why are you doing this? What do you want me to learn? To stay still and pay attention? Not to run around, run away? I am my body. I've always known that, as we all do primitively, but now it is clearer. Yet it is also clearer that I am not my body. My mind and spirit stand somewhat apart, able to analyze, ridicule, console. What a work we human beings are, my God. How inventive you have been in making us.

Why have you made us for ruin? I have so many questions for you, and yet prayer stops my mouth. Now and then it even stops my mind. When you embrace me, so that my spirit simply abides with you, my questions do not matter. You are all the answer I need.

The past few years I've thought from time to time about your femininity. What would it be like to enter your embrace as your lover? A delicate consideration, granted my sensuality and the history of Western spirituality. Yet a lovely possibility now, when I need you to be gentle, welcoming. I still want to move toward you. I still want to stand tall. If I cannot, do understand. As my physical strength diminishes, let me feel released rather than subjugated, drawn forward into you.

7. The Body and Jesus

Each day during chemotherapy I take more than twenty pills. I can't imagine what they are doing inside me. Some authors urge visualizing the good cells eating up the bad. When I try that I picture little creatures from pac-man games. It's hard to think that I am these processes, that they are changing me. People who live in their heads, even though they enjoy their bodies, know little about their cells.

I'm grateful for Jesus' emphasis on the spirit. You have given us myriad sacraments, O God, all illumined by your Word made flesh. The understanding of Jesus expressed in John's Gospel has always pleased me most: very God and very man. I do not understand those who shy away from Jesus' divinity. To safeguard his full humanity they go mute about his oneness with you, the absolute mystery. Surely that was settled hundreds of years ago, when canonical Christian faith insisted on both full humanity and full divinity. Surely we have no absolute savior, no absolute fulfillment of our humanity and history, if Jesus is no more than the best of our mortal kind.

Feeling completely mortal these days, I am greatly consoled by Christ on the cross. His vulnerability and courage would teach me all I need to know, were I faithful.

I also love the resurrected Lord in the Book of

Revelation, who makes all things new, including our mortal bodies. Earth has no full resonance without heaven. Jesus is not nonpareil, the unique place where we see the reaches of divine intimacy to our joint and marrow, unless he is God from God and Light from Light. Dying, he did not destroy our death, if he was not deathless as well as mortal. Rising, he did not give us deathlessness, divinization, unless he was the eternal Word breathing forth love.

I confess, God, my peasant, traditional understanding of Christ. I want, and need, your Christ to be all that the scriptures, councils, and creeds have proclaimed. He must be the Messiah, and even more the Son of God, with all the symphonic overtones such titles carry. He must be the Lord far above Caesar and so well worth dying for. I do not want to die for a religious hero, one savant among others. I want to die in union with, as a member of, your eternal self-image come into time as the most beautiful human being who ever lived, who ever could live.

8. Harboring High Hopes

Limping in spirit as much as body, how can I hope for healing, for peace, for salvation? Only because you promise them, my God. Only because you have sworn and cannot repent. I have no hope of salvation unless you are all that the scriptures proclaim. Without you, my life is barely a ripple of the cosmic wind. Yet I see you everywhere, feel you night and day, always knowing that you have to exist, if my desires are not a chimera.

The mere fact that I know I should be different and better, other people should be different and better, we should not have a Congress of fools, a church of bureaucrats, shouts that you have to exist. Where do my desires, the desires of any people of wit and good heart, come from, if not your Spirit? How can such desires be but the sport of monkey brains, the quirk of DNA?

Now that scientists think they have physical evidence of the first moments of creation and so can confirm the theory of the big bang, I hope that they will realize they have settled nothing. Why the big bang? Whence the explosion that set the entire mind-boggling drama of cosmic history going?

Certainly, this is not a scientific question, as we now define physical science. It is much more important than anything science can handle, anything science wants to handle. How strange that so many people are satisfied with intermediate answers and have no hunger for ultimate mysteries.

Christian faith forces us to rivet the big bang and everything else onto Jesus the Christ, the linchpin of the cosmos. All creation is in the Word, for everything that God is finds expression in the Word. And, as begun from a big bang, creation is much less than divinity. Divinity is all. Divinity plus creation is not more than divinity alone. Creation is divinity participated, partialized.

Dear God, I want you to be all in all. As I decrease day by day, I want you to increase in my wonder, my appreciation, my love. O God, my God, be everything to me. Even when my heart condemns me, be greater than my sins. I am not holy or worthy of you. Make it that I do not have to be. Save me despite myself, as another gratuitous work of your love. Show me, show the whole world, that you can carve something acceptable from the most flawed stone. Give glory to your own name, through my death.

9. Taking Care of Business

Today we got a new car. No longer will my wife drive her 1970 VW bug, bought new and treasured as the only car she's ever owned. Last week we bought a telephone answering machine. Soon we shall buy a color TV and VCR. My illness is moving us into the technological age most Americans have inhabited for a decade.

Dozens of other practical tasks impose themselves. There is insurance to review, a will to rewrite, the financial planning that prudence dictates. There are business deals and professional commitments that now have to be canceled. And there are all the medical contingencies: maybe a trip to a major clinic for a second opinion, maybe the need to contact the local hospice.

Much depends on how the chemotherapy proceeds. Unless it achieves a remission, I won't see the new year. Along with living day by day, one ache and challenge at a time, we have to face a future rushing toward us at indeterminate speed. Be, God, our balance. Have your Spirit keep us on an even keel.

Most important are our prayers, our sharing the beauties and pangs of this ordeal. Then come the nuts and bolts, the hieings off to doctors and lawyers, car dealers and insurance agents.

More and more the practical affairs fall to my wife. I used to do the dishes and some of the cleaning, most of the shopping, all the paying of bills and financial planning, most of the deals for the books we wrote. She earned most of our money as a university professor. It was a good arrangement, suiting us both. I was the dreamer with the mind for numbers. She was the teacher with the instinct for politics. Who are we now? What must she become for the future? I want time to work this out, dear God. I don't want to leave her unprepared. Maybe this is male protectionism to the end, but I ask you to let me get our affairs into good order.

Of course, if this is not to be, I have to let it go, along with everything else. But it would seem cruel to add practical problems to the emotional burdens Denise is sure to face. She'll be terribly lonely, in no shape to care about money or writing books. Again and again, you make it plain that dying is a series of renunciations. Some are physical: mobility, living free of pain. Some are things we planned: books, vacations, even conversations. Each day another set of images, another scenario for the future, falls into epoché.

Only you are certain, my God. Even my death has no date yet attached. So only you should preoccupy us. Ignatius Loyola thought it would take him fifteen minutes to reconcile himself to the dissolution of the Society of Jesus. Ignatius was detached, concerned only to do your will. Make us concerned only to do your will, my God. The rest is insignificant.

10. You Know Our Pain

My days are assuming some order, yet each day is different, if only because different physical symptoms arise. Yesterday the new phenomenon was edema, swelling in both legs and feet. Prescription: a diuretic, one little pill a day. Result: spectacular—about twelve cups of urine in twelve hours. No longer will I laugh at women who complain about monthly water retention. Have you hidden cisterns throughout our bodies, my God? Where does all this fluid hang out?

How much these changes in bodily fluids and other metabolic processes shape my thoughts and feelings is unclear. I now know that Tylenol 3, with its touch of codeine, makes a fecal cement that could seal peasant huts for a century. Serious sickness shows in piss and dung, as Chuang Tzu knew, as well as in pain and fear. All the better for an incarnational faith. All the more wonderful that you have taken flesh and dwelt among us, in order to know our sorrows and joys from within—the heart, the spleen, the bones.

From childhood I have prayed in churches dominated by a man hanging from a cross. "Who is that man, Mommy?" "That's Jesus, God's Son, who died because he loved us and wanted to save us from our sins." Accepting this as true, a child can grow up reconciled to death and pain. How brilliantly you have answered the problem of evil, my God. Beyond words, beyond understanding, you've shown that you know everything we suffer.

A suffering savior is the perfect response to our vulnerability. That your resurrected victor emerged on the far side of betrayal and death changes human existence exactly as it has to be changed, if we are to trust it, call it a profound comedy rather than a tragedy.

Accepting the message of the cross need not breed fatalism or contempt. The death and resurrection of Christ is the utter realism for which we human beings have been made. How deeply I feel that now, my God, when I ache to know you understand my suffering and pain. If I do not yet dare to contemplate triumph and resurrection, at least I know they are there, waiting for me to complete my preoccupation with passion.

You understand all that I fear, all that hurts me, as well as all that I hope, because you have feared, been hurt, had to fight to sustain your hopes. You, my God, seen in the countenance, heard in the voice, sensed in the broken bones of Jesus, your complete human icon, know all that I need. You are in me, with Jesus and your Spirit. The matter gone wrong in me, the pain that it causes, and the emotions spewn forth in consequence are patent to you as soon as they occur. You are more intimate to me than I am to myself. How could I exaggerate your goodness? Why should I ever feel alone?

11. I Am Tired

The chemical hits are taking their toll. I am tired but I still love to come to you for this new game, O God, with this new challenge. I am still awed by this new fact that I'm dying. But I have no strength for the blitz of emotions that this news, and then people's reactions, creates. Today's fatigue is like a quick transit from the sensual consolations of the early days of the spiritual life to the darker, dryer, probably more substantial work of the middle stages.

I do not need to feel you for you to be with me. I do not need to understand your ways for you to be wise, providential, fully in charge. Even the horror of losing my understanding, being driven into unconsciousness, is losing its force. If you need to take away my mind, so be it. I say that more bravely than honestly, because now my mind is my main defense against fear. But I have to begin to contemplate deeper losses. I have to begin to see that the offering you ask may be whole, a full holocaust.

Apocalypse is not the center of Christian faith, but the Book of Revelation is an irreplaceable gift. Reading it now, in tandem with the Psalms, consoles me mightily. The blazing beauty of the Lamb that was slain, the wonderful hymns of the elders before the throne of the one who was and who is and who is to come, quicken my spirit. What a tragedy that this book has become the playground of literalists and fundamentalists. How sad that few first-rate minds, apart from Ruysbroek, have fully exploited its white pebbles, its keys to death and Hades, its voice like the sound of rushing waters.

It is good for us to contemplate the end, from which you come to us. I think it likely that the parousia will be a bigger ontological bang than the creation of the physical universe.

O God, everywhere my mind goes you are consoling. If I rise to the highest heavens, you are there, resplendent in light. If I tumble toward the nadir of despair, you are there, your Son having suffered everything before me. Good God, my father, my mother, my all, it seems I cannot defeat you. You hunt me down. Not like a hound of heaven, but like the air I breathe, the spirit that makes me, the meaning that carries me into mystery at every turn.

No wonder the mystics go into unknowing. No wonder their minds shut down. We cannot say for sure, so we should simply abide. We cannot grasp you, so we should just love you—nakedly, comprehensively, exhaustively. Now you call me through fatigue to let go, just love. Now, beautifully, you make my tiredness into rest. The tears wetting my pillow are tears of joy. I may be going to you soon. It just might happen. You could be coming closer, pain by pain, fear by fear, to take me to yourself.

I can't really believe this yet, let alone presume it. But it is enough that it could be, that you let me hope it. At the depths of my soul, I've never wanted anything but you. Yet I've never felt I could be worthy of having this want, this hunger, this aching need fulfilled. Even after years of marveling at justification by faith, of loving the higher theology of grace that shows how you divinize us, how you give us your own trinitarian being, which is love, I find it hard to feel that you love me this way, that my mediocrity does not repulse you.

I know my feelings of unworthiness are common. One could write an entire theology of sin based on our inability to believe in your total goodness, starting with Adam and Eve ashamed of their nakedness. But that lessens none of the dynamite in my new hope that you are coming not to judge but to love. O felix cancer. If sickness convinces me of your love, makes me a credible witness to your utter goodness, it will be the best part of my life. My wife's love has prepared me for this, but only your palpable coming in the form of this terminal illness has brought my hope to crisis. Thank you, my God. I am not worthy that you should come under my roof, but only say the word and my dying will seem a pure grace.

12. When the Back Breaks

Early on the morning I was to begin a course of radiation on my back, my back broke. Coming out of the shower, I experienced a great fear that I would not be able to stand. Even with my wife's help I could not stand upright. Excruciating pain shot through my body and I tumbled back onto the bed. The pain was intense: I could find no place of support, no spot assuring me my back would not crack, my spine not snap.

I went by ambulance to the hospital but received no painkillers until the staff completed a battery of tests and determined my exact condition. For three hours I could only twist and writhe, finding a strange comfort in making mantras of my moans. I tried to offer these pains to you, my God, as you know, and to focus on the crucified Christ, but most of my energy went into enduring, simply surviving until I could receive analgesics to lessen the pain.

The first drug I received, demerol, was effective in deadening the pain, but soon I could barely distinguish between waking and dozing. Indeed, at times I was hallucinating: seeing things not physically present, shouting out parts of mental conversations I had been having silently (and so scaring my wife terribly). Switching to morphine brought a great improvement in my sense of reality, but for two or three days I was hard pressed to separate the imaginary from the physically real.

A full examination revealed that my myeloma was now manifesting itself through two crushed vertebrae and a large hole in my femur. Fearing a sudden pathological fracture caused by the weakness of the bone, my doctors wanted to operate while conditions were still relatively good, rather than deal later with the messiness of bones splintered or fractured by a fall.

The operation went utterly smoothly. I have no memory of becoming unconscious under the anesthesia, having the surgeons insert the pin and rod (a bloody, brutal procedure, I'm told), or coming back to consciousness. One moment I was in what seemed a small galley of a large operating room; the next moment I was in a recovery area, alert, able to converse, without significant pain. An hour later I was in my own private room, talking with my wife and two colleagues who had come to offer their support.

It will be six months, at least, before I regain anything like normal use of my right leg, but my experience of this operation has left me in awe of what surgeons now accomplish, apparently routinely. The helps available in a good hospital to anyone who is insured and able to pay would astound the most advanced scientists of the nineteenth century. Certainly they boggle my mind.

Seven weeks after a diagnosis of incurable cancer of the bone marrow, I have hosted chemicals, radiation, and physical manipulations I barely knew existed. Together these "guests" have taken away most of my pain, restored perhaps three-quarters of my physical energy, and allowed me to return to my work, which has become thinking about the religious (ultimate, metaphysical) implications of serious disease, both its effects on human beings and its possible revelations about divinity. You have taught me volumes about the Incarnation, my God. By lacerating my flesh, you have made your Christ a closer sacrament.

13. A Simple Prayer

The most helpful spiritual advice I've run across recently comes in a letter of "privy counsel" by the anonymous fourteenth-century Carthusian credited with *The Cloud of Unknowing*. The letter takes the core of his teaching on prayer and makes it utterly simple.

We need only adhere to you, dear God. We need only be before you, in you, with you, ideally in love, but even inertly, with no more feeling than a stone. You are our being, but so much more. More central than our thoughts or our feelings is your grant of existence, the love that makes us be. When we abide in our being, open to you, we rest in "hid divinity," to use another phrase of this master. So, when we feel the call, we should let go of all thoughts, worries, even joys that take us apart from you.

You call me to simplicity. I feel best when resting at my depths, on your buoyancy. Normally I have not felt, or accepted, the grace to be so simple. Normally my mind is distracted, my feelings squirt in a dozen directions. Now my body is teaching me stillness.

Last night the Jesus prayer came spontaneously, matching itself to my breaths. I did not sustain it long, but I recalled an Orthodox prioress who went into an operation saying the Jesus prayer and awakened from anesthesia still saying it. The prayer had taken over her respiration and heartbeat. Jesus had become her pulse.

The motif of the Letter to the Hebrews that we should enter the divine rest, your cosmic sabbath, has always pleased my soul. It offers the chance for a lovely balance. Inspiration and respiration. Systole and diastole. As you take over my being more physically, as I feel your gentle invasion, I breathe more lightly, more consciously, and sometimes more deeply.

The one yoga that has always drawn me is *pranayama*, breath control. Indian thought has long realized that breath joins matter and spirit. I pray now, God, for your Spirit, to take over my breath. I pray for your Son to make sacred the beats of my heart. And not, I hope, privately, in some pious or precious reprise of spiritualities past or sentimental. Possess me openly, socially, as a member of Christ's mystical body. Possess us all as branches of your vine.

14. A Last Good Day

Today may well be one of my last good days. I have no surety of tomorrow. Beyond the truth these sentences hold for any human being on any day, they should be the watchword of a cancer patient still uncertain of remission or anyone burdened by the cross of terminal illness.

The diet of phone calls and eulogies has become too rich. The waves of consolation threaten to swamp my bark. I am becoming more interested in what happens to me than in your primordial presence, my God. I am running far ahead, to dramatic consummations, while much tedious, commonplace trial and work may remain. Strangely, I am also forgetting the solid source of rightful intensity you offer me.

Without a remission, I probably have less than a year to live, perhaps much less. The median survival rate with remissions of multiple myeloma is about three years. So it is no hyperbole to greet each new day as one of a waning measure. I've got to become less adolescent, more mature about living before you unemotionally, more open to your movements in my heart.

I love the realism of many medieval mystics, fortunate to live in a pre-psychological time. We've learned reams from both later mystics and psychologists, but often we've lost simplicity and depth.

The early mystics remind us that our very existence is the primal mystery. That there is a world, rather than nothingness, remains the first wonder. If we are, O God, you must be, for we do not explain or ground ourselves. If you are, as you must be since we are, all things are possible. The wonders of grace, the magnificence of salvation history, paint these foundational truths in brilliant purples and oranges, delicate greens and rich reds. That you should be a perfect community of knowing and loving, that you should create to diffuse this consummate goodness, that you should recreate a world and people unthinkably ruined by sin — all this plays out the fullness of your goodness in technicolor. Eye has not seen nor ear heard a smidgin of the whole story.

But now, in my need for sobriety and minimalism, I want to bore into your quintessential being. I need darkness more than light. I want rest, being held, more than orgasm. Yet I should also want not what I want but what you want. I should also be wise enough to give you carte blanche. Who could care for me better?

15. Worry is Useless

Both John of the Cross and Teresa tell us not to be afraid. "Let nothing disturb you." When you hold me, or let me hold you, this otherwise incredible advice seems obvious. I live or die at your behest. I am merely another little grain of sand along the seashore, another twinkling star of Abraham's heaven. You move and rule all things sweetly, suavely. How we remain free to say yes or no to your movements, your love, is uncertain, though free we must be, if we are to become what you've made us.

I used to think that dying to live was a moral or paschal proposition. One put off the old person, as Paul suggested, to don the new. One went down with Christ in baptismal death and rose to trinitarian life. Now it is clearer that we do not do these things so much as undergo them. Now the primacy of your action, and the consequent primacy of our passion, stands forth. If there is any loss in my life that makes me reclaim it, better and fulfilled in you, that is your doing.

You work my death. All the little cells, cancerous or benign, strut their stuff at your behest. I can't begin to comprehend the nearly infinite delicacy and beauty of how you've arranged our cells and nerves. I understand none of the cytology or neurology, but the poetry soothes me. Often the metaphor seems musical. You are playing through us, circulating in our lymph. The harmonies of the spheres are echoing in our blood. Perhaps even the chorus of the 144,000 is sounding.

Along with gratitude for such a hope comes praise, the purest worship. The clearer we see, the more purely we feel, the more spontaneously we want only to praise you. For your beauty. For your goodness. For your mercy. The reasons or attributes multiply, but the core remains simple: for your being God. The mere, though hardly obvious, fact that you are God is enough. It alone makes our cup run over.

O God, be God for me, for all your people, for the whole world, today and everyday. Let us know, as you find best, that we are not alone and meaningless but a part of you, being of your Being. Plunge us into this overwhelming mystery, this ungraspable goodness and love, however we can best stand it, best profit from it. Do not be discouraged by our superficiality and our sin. Look to our hearts, our best desires, all the times and ways we hate being dirty and trivial. Show us, if only for a little while, that the impossible is possible: You could be for us. Christ could be, resurrected and saving. Love could be, from the beginning and unto all ages. Death could be your welcoming kiss.

16. Tools of the Trade

I am a writer by trade and even during my illness I have continued to work. My writing spot is decorated by a few spiritual reminders, some tools of my trade, and several nods to my cancer.

At my wife's request, one of our friends sent a crucifix, redeeming our atmosphere from complete paganism. He also sent a medal with Madonna and Child on one side and Ignatius Loyola on the other. Their familiar Jesuit ugliness comforts me. Receiving them from my friend recalls a friendship of over thirty years.

Two cards also lift my spirits. One is from the person who was to be my director for a thirty-day retreat. I've never met her, but the words she chose from Deuteronomy 31:8 pierce my heart day after day: "Don't be afraid, for God will go before you and will be with you." The other card is from a woman whose husband's bout with cancer several years ago was so courageous that I wrote a book about our conversations during his last days. Her card has a photo of a little kid, perhaps two, dressed in Oshkosh overalls, a red sweat shirt, and tiny sneakers. The kid (whether boy or girl is not clear) is struggling mightily to get a leg over the lowest rail of a country fence. The caption inside reads, "I know you can do it!" Every time I look at that little kid struggling I grin and feel my own determination harden.

For tools of my trade I have only a word processor

and a printer, a notebook, a few pens, an unabridged dictionary, a Bible, and a concordance of the New Testament. This project of coming to grips with a sentence of death is nothing scholarly. The main sources for accomplishing it lie within, in your darkness, my God. The main requisites are attention and unwonted honesty.

As bows to my illness I reckon a water bottle, a urinal, and, in the first weeks, a stack of kleenex for handling my uncertain emotions. Like a faithful dog, my aluminum cane waits patiently in the corner to help me haul myself up and stump off to new business.

Before me, most of the wall is blank. Within me, the tides change quickly. Sometimes all is calm, as blank as the wall. At other times everything roils. I feel your call in the calm, my God, but you must also be present in the upset. Give me, I pray, good work — not just distraction, something to keep my mind honed; rather an intellectual love of you that might help others laugh and suffer better. Let the humility of my little writing niche remind me how little space I deserve, compared to the great events, the truly significant sufferings and rebirths, proclaimed broadside in the *New York Times* each day.

What are my sufferings, my scribbles, my probably narcissistic hopes compared to the travails of the hundreds of thousands of people suffering throughout the world today? How wonderful that you are a God who deals with all of us personally, comprehensively. As is usually the case in Catholic theology, the right instinct

is both/and, not either/or. You are both the pan-
tokrator, the great Lord of cosmic history, and the beautiful, perhaps even shy lover of my soul. You are both
the unimaginable energy behind the Big Bang and the
still small voice soothing Elijah. My God, my God. You
never forsake us, never forget us, never are too busy to
notice our needs. To the end of my days I will praise
you. If you keep sending your Spirit, I shall keep wanting only your honor and glory.

17. Coping with Visitors

I did not want visitors in the hospital and I've not been hospitable to them since I've returned home. In the hospital, the combination of chemotherapy, radiation, and the major operation on my leg had pushed my blood counts alarmingly low. This necessitated my being isolated from ordinary hospital traffic. The staff kept visitors to a minimum, and anyone dealing with me—doctor, nurse, even my wife who was sharing my room—had to wear a protective mask.

I have always loved solitude and disliked crowds, thrived in quiet and been irritated by noise. It was a perverse blessing that I should be so weak as to draw from a hospital—always a busy, potentially noisy place—its maximal provision of isolation. When I felt strong enough, I read spiritual books and wrote in a diary. I discussed all species of things, funny and grim, with my wife. One session, we might focus on financial planning, in view of the contingency that my terminal illness could soon make her a widow. Another time we might discuss the image of Jesus in the first chapters of Mark's Gospel, where he bursts on the scene as a powerful healer.

My interior life showed a similar diversity. Sometimes I prayed effectively, losing myself in the mystery of your will, O God. At such times, deep in my consciousness, there seemed to sound, like a drum from the Congo forest, the reminder that I would live or die, secure a remission or worsen to critical status, as you chose. Doctors, drugs, and I myself were all playing important roles in how my disease unfolded, but ultimately this terminal illness would proceed as it had begun: at your impenetrable behest. Other sessions of prayer, as you know, were as superficial and distracted as I often suffered long before I became ill.

The hospital was not good at dealing with the ultimate dimension of disease, the mysteriousness expressing your divine sovereignty. My doctors did not mention it, though clearly they were aware of their limitations and recognized that more than biological factors have much to say about human illness or health.

Some of my nurses, moved by evangelical fervor, spoke much of the Lord's will. But, understandably (granted our secular, pluralistic American culture), the mysterious origins and destiny of my terminal illness remained something left to me, the patient, to understand. This conspiracy of silence about ultimate matters amused me, indeed consoled me, even when I felt sad that I did not live in a time or culture where the agencies of the divine and human could move together harmoniously.

Granted the mysteriousness of how divine freedom sustains human freedom, perhaps no time or culture has ever been able to comfort the sick thoroughly at all levels of their confusion and hurt. Still, I long for opportunities to clarify how vigorously I ought to work and pray for a remission. I am eager to dialogue with people who will understand if I say it might be a blessing of God for me not to gain a remission. I want a remission. I want to live and to return to robust health, in good part because I feel my love of life reflects the judgment of the God of Genesis that creation is very good. But perhaps you have a deeper wisdom.

I am haunted by the massive uncertainty at the center of my situation. No one can tell me how I will be feeling a year from now—if there is then any me. To be sure, this uncertainty applies to all people's lives. Indeed, it is virtually a definition of the human condition. But now, in my case, the uncertainty of the future has narrowed to seemingly specific yet actually unpredictable factors such as blood counts, the production of plasma in my bone marrow, and my response to cytoxin and other lethal chemicals.

Early in the morning and late at night, my guardian angel carries me to these thoughts. The ultimate causality I both love and fear has no place in the charts recording every medication I receive, every bowel movement I produce. Still, your hand and will are far more significant. At the end of my thoughts, as in the beginning, darkness prevails. It is the dominant spiritual medium as night after night, your Spirit broods over waters too primeval for me to sound.

18. Abandonment

The lesson I'm hearing today concerns abandonment.
You make a chorus, if not a single voice, of the *Cloud*,
John of the Cross, Teresa, Brother Lawrence, and de
Caussade. I hear them telling me that my life is your doing, as my being is your giving. The more I give my life
and death, my self and being, over to you, the better for
everyone. Who knows what is true living and good dying? You alone. Socrates going to his death remains a
consoling figure: Arguably he was doing a far, far better
thing than the senators who condemned him.

Should I pray for a remission, if the price would be a
lesser death? Have I even the right to ask this question?
The question fades when abandonment takes center
stage. I should pray for what will most honor you, what
you know is best for me, and for all for whom I'm responsible.

My complete instinct is that you control my fate. I
can't conceive of suicide, though of course much may
change and many people face death in circumstances
different from mine. Still, opposing suicide seems to imply fighting hard to preserve the physical life you've giv-
en me.

I'm amused, but also pleased, that my body takes
chemotheraphy as a challenge. Maybe it's due to boy-
hood sports and years of hard exercise, including one
very slow marathon. Whatever the causes, I find my

body quickened and engaged. Even when I lie down exhausted, I feel in the midst of a good fight, a competition of which to be proud.

All the more is this the case with my mind and spirit. At the risk of shocking some people, I have to confess, my God, that I love what you're asking. I don't love the pain or the real threat of dying. I hate the burden I've become to myself and Denise, to my family and many friends. But I love the challenge you've issued me. You've raised the ante so high that even I can't miss the significance. You've promoted me to the big show, the major league.

Sometimes I think I see the point to the classical description of the love of wisdom (philosophy) as the practice of dying. Now and then it occurs to me that this cancer is my passover, my *kairos*, my individual *eschaton*.

19. Battling Death

Like a cocky bantamweight, I want to jump into the ring and begin my battle with death. I've yet to reckon with the possibility that in the other corner may stand Jack Dempsey, the Manassa Mauler. I've no idea how cruel or ugly Sister Death may turn out to be. My faith denies that she can become Kali, the goddess who loves bloody destruction, whose signature jewelry is a garland of skulls. But I'm a fool if I assume death must be sweetness and light.

Until now I've never suffered great physical pain. I have no idea what toll aching, throbbing, hurting to one's bones day after day may exact. Again, my God, I pray for sobriety, minimalism, balance. "In the midst of consolations, remember your past desolations, and prepare to be tested again." Good advice from a long line of Christian spiritual masters, though perhaps not so necessary as its complement: "In the midst of desolations, believe God will return to console you, as God always has done in the past."

I thank you now, my God, for your many consolations, recent and longstanding. What more could you have done for me, for any of us? The sins that have kept me from serving you well are cause for more than blushing. Yet now you push me toward a deeper humility, letting me feel your complete sovereignty over my whole being, letting me rejoice that your will is what will be, if I only say yes.

My delight should be to give you free reign. Many masters of prayer say nothing pleases you more than our trust. I do want to trust you. I do want to pay attention, focus on you more than myself, or my work, or my ambitions, or even my fears. "You are a good God, and you love our kind," says a wonderful Orthodox prayer. I love your kindness, my God, the mercy that grounds my hope. If you count my failures, I have no hope.

If I count your blessings, heaven stands wide open. Indeed, there, worthy as the Lamb that was slain, Jesus assures me that those who keep faith, who cling to you in trust, see your goodness unveiled, and so join the seraphim and cherubim in offering you ceaseless praise. I want to be there, my God, in that chorus of praise. I want to offer you ceaseless admiration, and so I pray: Make my dying an acceptable passport. Take me to your promised land, far across the Jordan, far beyond my best imaginings, where you dwell in inestimable light, the God from whom all good things descend.

20. *Poisoning Myself*

I'm going off to poison myself. Deliberately, I'm going to kill cells in my body, many of them healthy and good. The hope, of course, is that I shall kill more cells that are sick and destructive. Such is the course of treatment known as chemotherapy.

I marvel at the courage of medical scientists, as well as their brilliance. They are willing to grapple with the mechanisms of living and dying on a daily basis. Perhaps some of them do like to play God, but the ones I've come to know during this illness are humble about their limitations. Indeed, I see great faith in their ability to do what they can and leave the rest to what they might call fate.

My oncologist has consistently been cheerful, full of hope without offering a shred of illusion. What went into his choice of this specialty? What must it take to deal every day with terminal patients, humanity brought into extremis? Something priestly attends his demeanor. He stays away from spiritual advice in his instructions, yet always seems aware that cancer is more than physical. A touch of the freedom that the dying themselves can enjoy moves in the air around him. He seems to feel privileged to work at something ultimate, something heightening human significance, even though often the daily phenomena, the brutally physical facts, are grim.

I was seeking this privilege when I began college by signing up for pre-med. The lure of ultimacy thrilled me and frightened me, when early in my schooldays I witnessed a car accident that sliced open a woman's leg. Someone would have to put all that bloody spaghetti back in order. What skill and courage he or she would need! I never learned whether I would have had the courage. Since I kept ruining dogfishes in biology class it seemed clear to me that I did not have the skill.

Some of that first shudder and thrill still runs down my back when I enter a hospital, especially an emergency room. Perhaps the emotional jolt of finding an analogous drama now occurring in my own body accounts for much of my fascination. Even though I feel drawn to stress spiritual combat more than physical, I am deeply impressed by the sheer facticity of the bodily dimension, and long to tie them to faith. Because Jesus ached in his bones, even the most obvious of my symptoms are Christian. If Jesus healed bodies as well as minds and hearts, the most basic of my doctors' ministrations are messianic. All of this cancer, as all of the social impact it brings to and from other people, is full of your glory. Strange, strange. Wonderful, wonderful.

21. Enduring Pain

Family members and friends forced to watch a loved one suffer through a serious illness naturally wonder about the intensity of the pain. Patients themselves are, perforce, equally concerned with pain, though usually with less wonder and more resignation.

Before describing physical pain, as I have come to know it at new levels during this terminal illness, let me thank you, my God, for what seems a psychological mercy you have built into our humanity, the union of matter and spirit that comprises our selves. We—at least I—cannot remember past pain except generally, vaguely: "terrible;" "like a knife;" "a bone-deep ache." Those words may seem concrete, reason to recoil, but they barely suggest what the lived experience of the pain actually was.

We are unable to reproduce emotions based primarily in bodily disorders, especially horrible ones, except in such general terms that recalling them does not wipe us out or force us never to risk such pain again. When pain is persistent and patterned, as were the muscle spasms that became my cross during the first weeks in the hospital, each new pain fits itself into the ongoing pattern and so seems frighteningly familiar. Nonetheless, even an hour's freedom from muscle spasms (there were periods when I had one every fifteen minutes) lessens one's fears, begins to blur the sharp features of the memory, and so allows one to escape feeling like a feral prisoner.

If you had not given us this strange amnesia or incapacity, my God, the lives of those suffering painful physical sicknesses would be hellish, as in fact are the lives of those who can get no relief from their physical pains, either because no analgesic can touch them or because their bodily system has so broken down that no mechanisms of relief remain. For such people, I can only pray, shuddering, and beg others to pray similarly. Why have you abandoned some of your children to agony, my God? Please hasten, rush with all heavenly speed, to take them to yourself, into your heaven, and wipe every tear from their eyes. Otherwise, you will seem sadistic.

22. Reducing Pain

I knew going into the hospital that I was no hero, likely to bear pain stoically, with neither outburst nor other sign of concession. My only goal was to survive, to manage to get through. So sometimes I screamed, and sometimes I winced. Therapists taught me how deep breathing can lessen pain. Habituation made me tougher. But I remain an opponent of pain, a man who dislikes being hurt. I am a kindred spirit to Job, wondering why God has put so much pain and injustice into creation and history.

Much as I hope that I will not need techniques such as controlled breathing in the future, realism suggests that I shall, so I keep working on them. Sometimes, when the breathing is going optimally, I become one with the pain in such a way that it diminishes considerably. For a time it seems to be a part of me, rather than a foe frightening me from the outside. I move with the pain and work through it rather than fighting against it. I relax, and thereby narrow the target I offer the spasmic muscles (or the devil manipulating them). I have learned not to follow my natural reflex to stop breathing and not to resist this ugly intruder, since that only subjects my whole body to greater suffering. Combined with effective drugs, good breathing has cut my physical sufferings and my brutal bodily pains considerably (certainly in half). Even before radiation destroyed major sources of such suffering, breathing deeply and regularly had helped greatly to reduce my suffering.

I know only a beginner's amount about pain, fortunately, and a beginner's amount about how best to approach it or slide away from it. But even this beginner's quotient is enough, my God, to make me tax you with every suffering person's question: "Why must we undergo such pain?" Night or day, I get no answer.

As soon as I raise this question I find myself pondering Christ on the cross with renewed incomprehension. For us human beings and our salvation—for me, specific, spotty, spasmatic me—Christ emptied himself, dying in horrible physical pain on a cross like a slave. For me he was cursed and suffered the fate of a heinous criminal. For me he was tempted to think he was abandoned by you, his beloved Father, because you seemed to do nothing to rescue him. Greater love than this I cannot conceive, even though the necessity for it continues to escape me.

Once and for all, I gather, you wanted to show us that you have identified your very being with our humanity. You wanted to prove that nothing human is foreign to you, save sin. Silently, with the eloquence of a deed that a million words could never match, you showed us that you have known suffering so intimately that, in consequence, it has been fractured, broken to bits, and, like death, lost its sting. Let it be, God, let it be.

23. Finding My Way to God

I think I've found my prayer, and so my way. I want to be with you, my God, as simply and comprehensively as possible. I want my heart to speak to your heart, my being to cling to your being, far below the level of mind or emotions, in a colloquy or embrace of the love that makes you you and me me. The author of *The Cloud of Unknowing* has reminded me of the spirituality I've always most loved: spare, apophatic, adamantine— yet liquid with love.

The past days have been too rich. This morning I felt like I did many years ago, after I had hurtled down the slide at the neighborhood park. Dumped on the ground, breathless, shaking my head free of dizziness, I began to put one dusty foot in front of the other, in an effort to make dying plodding, ordinary. No more theater, God, unless you open a new show. Enough with romantic scenarios. A new motto: Sufficient for the day is the evil thereof. Will I be willing, able, to accept this discipline?

Formidable indeed are my unbridled mind, my self-satisfaction, my enjoyment of singular status. Part of me likes being special, standing out from the crowd. I find myself conceding to the awkwardness of others and so making cancer into business as usual, even comedy. To be sure, some of this is healthy. You want us to de-mythologize the principalities and powers. Yet some of my collusion in distraction is also cowardly. Teach me the difference between minimalism and distraction, and give me the guts to honor it.

I find being unusual strange, and so have much to learn about how to use my peculiar kind of privilege ("he has bone cancer, you know") to make other people more thoughtful. I don't want to become sententious or self-important. Yet, even more, I don't want to turn my back on the gift you have made me. You have forced me to think of each day as one of a dwindling few. On all sides, friends and acquaintances need to hear this message. I'd like to get it under their skin without being too irritating. Otherwise, I'm just another bit of news, flashy today but ignorable tomorrow.

More than my pride is hurt when the reality of my condition is ignored. Hurt as well is the core of Christ's message: "The time has come. The Kingdom of God is at hand. Repent, and believe in the good news." Yes, the fate of Christ's message, the acculturation of the gospel, is a perverse comfort, as well as a continual horror. If they have disregarded the Master who died and rose for them; if even he has become old news; what should I expect but quick relegation to familiarity and innocuousness? No servant is greater than his Master, can avoid his Master's fate.

Perhaps I can step out of line on occasion and remind those who think they have me pegged that only a few protein cells separate their good health from my moribundity. It can be fun to make mischief, not be the good little boy, the respecter of people's sensibilities. By being open about my illness I can challenge society's insistence that God and death stay completely private. The more I think that way, my God, the more interesting future social interactions become.

Jesus upset the scribes and pharisees. Jesus was unpredictable. And Jesus is my model, the sacrament of how I want to live and die. So, I have the perfect theological rationale for being mischievous. Not only can I ward off boredom, I can reflect some of the provocation of my Master — as long as I don't get too clever or self-satisfied.

The simple prayer that has dealt best with my cancer tosses peripheral things to the side. Like Thomas Aquinas summing up his tomes, I find myself thinking, "It's all straw." What I've done, for good or evil, matters little. You, God, have made all things new. You can redeem my life from the pit. If today I hear your voice, and do not harden my heart, I can praise you in the assembly of your saints, as you deserve. If I avoid the grumblings of my forebears at Meribah, I can enter your promised land.

The first of Bernard Lonergan's marvelous transcendental precepts comes to mind: Be attentive! Stop your wandering. Quiet your shiftless imagination and watch, wait, abide. Don't be like the disciples in the Garden. Don't give in to your usual torpor. Your adversary, like a circling lion, longs for you to lower your guard. Grow complacent and he'll eat you for lunch. The beginning of wisdom is fear of the Lord. The desert fathers knew all the rules of combat. Take a lesson. Don't be a fool, as you have been so often in the past.

24. An Anointing

It was a slow Sunday afternoon when a local priest whom I admire as a genuine pastor ambled into my room. He delivered himself of a few stories, his equivalent of small talk, and then asked what priests had been visiting me. I laughed and reported that spiritual ministrations had been minimal. Irritated, but not surprised, he asked if I would like to be anointed. With no thought, I said yes. So we went through a spare, adapted version of the Church's ancient ritual that asks God's help for the seriously sick—begs divine support and comfort for both body and spirit. Although it began almost shamefully casually, this anointing proved to be the most moving moment in my month's stay in the hospital. Indeed, it has lodged itself among the half-dozen most moving religious experiences of my entire life.

When I took religious vows as a Jesuit, I thought my future would run as straight as a pair of railroad tracks. When I was ordained a priest, I knew my future would be hopelessly tangled, because I had lost faith in the Church's rules about celibacy. In both cases, though, I assumed that I had time, that things would sort themselves out, that the wilderness could prove habitable, the desert could bear fruit.

Lying in my narrow hospital bed, feeling the oil of gladness and healing, I knew I had little time. More importantly, though, I felt, by your wondrous grace, that this was the first time in my effective memory that the Church, in the representative figure of one of its priests (who, at a still deeper level of representation, stood for Christ), was praying for me individually, by name, to deal with painful circumstances, suffering, and needs uniquely my own.

Even writing this description of what must have been at most ten minutes of unpretentious prayer moistens my eyes, as the anointing itself did in abundance. I realized, on my hospital pallet, that "Mother Church" had not been my mother for a long time. Psychologically (not theologically), Mother Church had kicked me out, waived visiting rights, and said the divorce from my role as "father" (due to my independent convictions about love and Christ) suited her fine. In a dozen ways Mother Church shouted that I was a big disappointment. Through the twenty-odd years of estrangement my typical response, usually thrown imaginatively toward the tubby clergy claiming to represent Mother Church, was a simple Italian hand gesture, bawdy and amused.

Anointing was a very different business. Something maternal really did appear. I felt taken to the bosom of a holy mother, a loving family that cared for me. It knew about my muscle spasms and dismal prognosis. It loved me despite my manifest failings and my worst sins. And it dismissed the past history, the tubby clerics, the mutual antagonism and disappointment of mother and child, as irrelevant.

For once, the church did not point to itself but was transparent to God. For once it was a community of prayer, offering the praise and petition that have always been its primary reason to be. And, for what seemed to me the first time, I, little John, weak John, competent John, mixed-up John, strong John, very sick John had a name in this community. My pain aggrieved it. My dying would sadden and diminish it. I mattered. For once, I mattered.

I still can't get over the power in this feeling or perception of mattering, of being an irreplaceable individual. Where the late bishop of Wichita had told me and my wife not to come to live in his diocese, because we would not be welcome, the church at prayer in my anointing said, "Welcome home. Forget that asshole."

Where the Roman authorities, in granting my dispensation from priestly celibacy to marry, had told me to move five hundred miles away, not teach theology, and not worry about my illegitimate children because the dispensation automatically legitimated them (in fact, my wife and I have no children), the church at prayer in my anointing said, "We ask God, who is wholly good, to strengthen your body and spirit, for we love you and care about you, as God does infinitely more. We are not clerics, bureaucrats, bloodless functionaries. We are your family, your brothers and sisters, mortal and sinful like you, sure one day to need anointing ourselves. Come close, into our embrace. Become part of the communion of saints as we intercede for you with God. Be at peace."

I know that terminal illness can throw people for emotional as well as physical loops. I know that on that Sunday afternoon I was susceptible to a great range of feelings. But I also know, with far greater certainty, that my anointing that day was the most sacramental experience I've had in a long time, the most healing and edifying. Blessings on that good priest who wandered in because of the radar that good priests develop. Blessings on all the Christians through the centuries who have sustained the sacrament of the sick. And, above all, blessings on you, Mother Church, for showing me, if only for a little while, that your maternity is more than rhetorical.

Part Two

25. A Cycle of Chemotherapy

A year dominated by chemotherapy offers interesting lessons in the ways and vulnerabilities of the body. The six different cancer-killing chemicals that I took became familiar invaders with predictable effects. The first few days of the month-long cycle (when I was actually taking the drugs) tended to speed up my engine and shorten my sleep. For the next several days of the cycle I often found myself tired, irritable, and longing to stop taking the drugs. I felt full of chemicals—my body bloated, my taste buds tainted.

The week following the intake was usually the worst. Withdrawing the prednisone, along with starting to feel the "hit" of the other chemicals in my marrow, tended to cause aching, fatigue, and susceptibility to migraines. I could not be sure that I would be able to work. Social obligations were a welcome distraction, but sometimes I would find it hard to concentrate, because of fatigue. Weeks three and four tended to be better—sometimes nearly normal, sometimes only dogged by fatigue. Inevitably, though, the chemotherapy dominated my horizon, especially during the early months, when I was still learning its patterns.

I am grateful that my physical reactions were seldom hard to endure. I never experienced the heavy nausea that depresses some cancer patients, tempting them to quit. More often than not I could smile at the aching bones or the tiredness that would sweep in. I've had migraines most of my life. Those induced by the withdrawal of the drugs presented no new problems, just the old challenge to resign myself and go to bed.

I found that I did better combating the effects of the chemotherapy by exerting myself, working as hard as I could, rather than by babying myself. Sometimes I would have to quit, but more often than not I got stronger if I tried to push through the fatigue.

During the week when I was actually taking the drugs, I would usually rise about four A.M., convinced that I could sleep no more (by then I would have been at least half-awake for two hours), and go to work. It would be dark and quiet, ideal for concentrated thought. Early morning has always been my most creative time. On occasion the chemicals seemed to enhance my creativity. Indeed, during the last of my cycles I did the first draft of a 250-page book in two weeks, riding the charge of the prednisone. I just kept working away, ignoring the fatigue as long as I could and shutting down for a few hours when I could not. I was so pleased to be getting large handfuls of work done that I almost welcomed the next dose of drugs.

Strange are your ways, O God of our bodies and time. Different than we expected are the paths of righteousness along which you lead us.

26. Chemotherapy and God's Will

When my oncologist suggested stopping the chemotherapy, I saw more clearly another dimension of how I had been coping. Going to his office for the thirteenth treatment, I had expected another six months in which to prepare myself psychologically for the cessation of our war on the cancer, and for the advent of what I pictured as the second phase of the venture, when we waited for the myeloma to rise from the canvas and begin battling again.

Stopping early, after twelve rather than eighteen month-long sessions, speeded up my process of psychological adjustment. Presto, the safety net had been snatched away and I was working the high wire with nothing to catch me. Actually, I knew that if the cancer were to start growing again, we could return to chemotherapy, but my initial sense of stopping was that I was losing a key defense mechanism.

The religious challenge of this situation brought a new spate of images. God seemed to become more immediately involved in my survival. The will of God became manifest in the cellular processes occurring in my body. I saw the rise and fall in the serum protein electrophoresis counts as imprints of the hand of God. Images of free-fall threatened, with only the will of God, your embrace, to catch me.

Of course, deeper reflection reminded me that we always fall into the hands of the living God. We never live by anything more intimate, ultimate, or decisive than your will. If you choose, a bolt of lightning or a truck hurtling round the corner can end any life abruptly, whether or not the person is undergoing chemotherapy. No therapy defends us from the general vulnerability lurking in the bones and circumstances of all living things, all citizens rural or urban.

People of faith, moreover, ought to believe that God's disposition of their days serves their benefit. None of us knows the day or the hour of our demise, and that in itself is good, because it invites all of us to stay alert, seize the day, pay attention. None of us knows whether a long life would be more beneficial to our salvation than a short life. All of us have to trust that how our time unfolds, what God chooses to number as the sum of our days, is to our advantage.

Specifically, I have had to convert my mind to the proposition that contracting cancer of the bone marrow in the fifty-third year of my life was a gift from God. Certainly, it is a strange gift, challenging and paradoxical. Nonetheless I need to view it as being for my good, and perhaps for the good of others. Otherwise, God does not number my days for my benefit. Otherwise, God does not redeem our time, write straight with crooked lines, prove wiser than our human estimates of prosperity.

27. Feeling Good Again

At the moment, I do not feel threatened by death. I have recovered a large portion of my pre-cancer health, perhaps eighty-five percent, and can work fairly normally. I do not writhe in pain. My temperamental inclination not to worry has held up, keeping depression away.

As my illness takes its course I see much benefit in imagining that God is disposing my time quite intimately. It feels properly religious to think this way, and it seems to bind me closer to God. I sense the workings of the divine Spirit more finely. I pray more simply and feel more intensely that I am convenanted to God and should let God travel with me day by day.

Has God a stake in my shift to a more naked encounter with my illness? Does God want this new phase of my little drama to occasion closer contact, fuller intimacy? I cannot know God's mind, but my faith suggests that this could be so.

Simply accepting the fact that I have a terminal disease tends to sharpen my mind and sketch the proportions of my life more clearly. Medical procedures, however, can dull the impact of my illness and cloud the stark reality that I may be dead soon. I need to strike a balance between reliance on human healing activities and my trust in the Lord.

In this regard, I have thought several times of Ignatius Loyola and Francis of Assisi, both of whom felt drawn to a strict poverty. As they tried to discern God's will for their religious orders in regard to the vow of poverty, they both wanted the least possible reliance on human means of support, so as to magnify their followers' trust in God's providence.

The analogy for those of us invaded by terminal illness depends on both our circumstances and how God's Spirit seems to move in our depths. Certainly, we ought to use the medical helps that our doctors encourage. God expects us to honor both human intelligence and the regular laws of nature. On the other hand, when we are thrown more nakedly, more directly, upon the divine will, we can tell ourselves that this has the benefit of engaging our faith more profoundly. Then, whether our health prospers or fails can seem to be the will of God immediately, directly.

All along, of course, God uses both our actions and the actions of natural agents to fulfill the divine purposes, execute the divine plan. But it can be well for us to think that we are bypassing intermediaries and receiving God's immediate influence. It can be well for us to pray again as we did in the beginning, when we first glimpsed what it means to be a mortal creature: "Come God, my death (or my life). Do with me what you will, what the love of your heart prompts. Help me to trust that this has to be good."

28. Good Friends

Denise and I have had wonderful support from our friends, and we have learned some important lessons from them. For the most part, our friends have stayed faithful, calling or writing us regularly. In a few cases, my sickness seems to have become old news, so that a friend's old habits of busyness or ambiguous, complicated emotions have rendered communication sporadic.

People dealing with a terminal illness regrettably report that their friends vary in how they handle the news, in what they will and will not let the illness mean to them. Cancer carries special overtones, special fears, tending to provoke more dramatic reactions than less threatening illnesses.

The majority of our best friends are religious, but we are close to a fair number of people who neither go to church nor are comfortable with religious language. I have been pleased that not all of our friends are Catholics, or Christians, or even religious people. That has seemed to suggest that we need not live in a ghetto, that the wide world of plain humaneness has a place for us. On the other hand, there is a depth of sharing, an intimacy of understanding, hard to achieve without agreement on fundamental, bedrock issues, among which matters of faith are paramount.

I feel a new bond with a Jesuit priest, now quite aged, who was my teacher and spiritual director many years ago. Age has brought him into the same realm of the spirit, the same zone of destiny, that terminal illness has brought me. We are both conscious that quite probably time is short, the judgment of God is near. Of course, both of us may survive quite a few more years, but we would be foolish not to be preparing our spirits. I will visit him soon and our prospective conversation intrigues me. Ideally it will cut across the ten years or so since we last met and deal directly with death and the other great mysteries we face.

The friends who have been most apparently, overtly faithful have found ways, often quick and small, to keep in close touch. One busy man, a college president, sends postcards almost weekly. Often they present paintings by Matisse, his passion of the moment. He tends to write them on the fly, as he moves around the country. I know that keeping some form of priestly ministry is important to him, and I am delighted that he has found so efficient and effective a means. He only writes four or five lines, yet they convey volumes of interest, care, and prayerful support.

A few other friends call on a regular basis, perhaps once a month, as though a wake-up alarm goes off if they have not had direct contact with us for a while. I am grateful that they feel it necessary to make contact and want to sustain familiarity.

I think this way myself, tending to regularize the relationships that I consider crucial or desirable. For example, Denise and I now write a one-page report every three months, a period that seems a natural measure for informing stockholders of how their investment is going. I call a few fellow-sufferers of serious illness every month or so, to keep tabs on the course of their cancer or Alzheimer's disease.

I call my mother weekly, because that seems both to keep her fears low and give her pleasure. She has just celebrated her eightieth birthday, and though she is slowing down, her health is much better than mine. One of the benefits of my taking sick has been her sharing in it, which has brought us closer than we had been. Though not estranged, we had had no reason to talk seriously or work at bridging the gap in our generations. Now we have a solid reason, and we have used it well.

The friends who have supported us best are those who in their distinctive ways make it clear that they love us. It is impossible to have too many people telling you persuasively, not just as a matter of course or at the end of a boozy evening, that they love you. You still have to take what they say with a grain of salt, but you can chalk it up to their goodness and neither blush nor dismiss it wrongly.

Sick people of any sensitivity soon find that they have to let themselves be cared for, worried over, exalted beyond their merits—in a word, loved. That is part of the job description of being sick, especially of being sick terminally. Your fate reminds all who see you that they also are mortal. Your fate becomes a nutshell in which the pathos of the entire human condition rests.

Finally, people suffering from terminal illnesses also have to resist the pressure to present a countenance heroic or pious or wise. You have to fight hard to be yourself, put on no airs, but also take no guff. Whatever you can do to remind people that illness is a regular part of life, nothing extraordinary, is a gift to them. No matter how healthy they are now, most of the friends who come to visit will eventually be more like you than different. Whatever you can do to make trust in God, agreement to what God makes happen, seem natural and easy will be a blessing.

29. God Caused This

God is the source of my cancer. I cannot avoid this conclusion, if I want to retain a biblical faith, in which not
a hair of our heads goes unnumbered, not a sparrow
flies unremarked. Admittedly, the Jesus who used this
example to indicate God's care for all of creation did
not live in the modern world shaped by a physical science that stresses secondary, intermediate causes.
Admittedly, I believe in evolution, and I believe as well
that the natural sciences deserve full autonomy in describing how evolution (in the widest possible sense of
the history of the natural world) seems to have unfolded. I solve the merely apparent problem of wanting
to hold such contemporary positions while also holding
a biblical trust like that of Jesus by noting that in any
proper theological scheme, biblical or contemporary,
God is the ultimate cause of everything that exists. To
deny that proposition would be to deny the reality of
"God," either merely mouthing traditional words or re-
ducing divinity from the infinity that biblical faith associates with it to something limited.

A limited God is no God, if the measure of divinity is
traditional biblical, patristic, and conciliar faith. If I
wish to retain a traditional faith, I must make God the
ultimate source of my cancer. In similar fashion I need
to see God as the ultimate cause of the floods that wreak
havoc when a river overflows its banks, the hurricanes

that devastate the American south, and the AIDS viruses that pass from addicted mothers into children in the womb.

Jesus knew that his God was responsible for his crucifixion, yet his faith never buckled under this burden. He commended himself into his Father's keeping, although perhaps he could not understand, in that part of his being where his workaday mind functioned, why his Father should require such suffering.

I cannot understand the plan of God, the necessity that there be evil, the law of the cross that stipulates that we only overcome evil by suffering it in love. These things are too great for me, too heavy.

But we human beings can endure such things, can accept them, can even love them, to the extent that we can see them as dispensations of the God who ravishes our hearts with her beauty, secures all our hopes with his fidelity. Apart from a God who makes all things new, who can redeem our lives from the pit of death or innocent suffering, and who can be greater than our hearts even when our hearts condemn us, the world becomes horribly absurd. If the real, living, always greater God is dead, anything, everything is permitted. All bets are off, no rules are grounded, sanity swings free of its moorings and becomes an ape, ready to serve whoever offers the best banana.

30. The Pain of Friendship

The friends who have given us pause, caused us pain, are those who have ignored the change in our circumstances. In the measure that we had felt close to them, involved with them, we had given them the power to hurt us. Some, unfortunately, have exercised that power, though usually largely unawares.

You expect your close friends to pay attention to your moods, be interested in the details of your sufferings, care about your ups and downs. You expect them to support you, because, you like to think, you would support them, care about them, be alert and pay attention to their needs, were the shoe on the other foot. That is what friends do, how love comports itself. When that is not what people do, you find yourself forced to re-evaluate the friendship. And you resent this.

You should not have to wonder where you stand with people who call themselves your friends. You know that your needs would bulk larger than their busyness or fears or perverse regrets that their lives are not so dramatic as yours, if they were in fact good friends. Thus, your mental printer tends to become revisionist, spewing out a new version of your history with these people that brands your past interpretation of the friendship as deluded.

I do not know what to make of friends who fail to come through or who give no support when the time of crisis arrives and the issue is truly one of life or death. I feel much as I feel when I must deal with genuine sin, either in others or in myself. I find myself confronted with a core irrationality, something that makes no sense, and I can only accept it with pain and tears of regret.

We fallible, distractable, fragile human beings have to forgive one another our liability not to come through in the crunch when people ask us to stand up and be counted. The commonplace reality is that we can become inured to tragedy, used to pain, bored by a friend's terminal status. The commonplace truth is that we can both be too weak to handle a friend's trouble, because it exposes our own mortality, and pleased that he or she has come into crisis while we continue to be healthy.

It does not profit people who are suffering to prolong their forays into the pathologies of friendship, but bare realism suggests that, when evidence of such pathology presents itself, we must not blink it away. When a friend fails us, we can take another lesson in the frailty of human nature, in the sole adequacy of God. Such a failure is bound to hurt us, but if it threatens our religious faith we have not been believing well. Jesus had to endure the desertion of Judas, as well as the lesser flight of ten of the remaining twelve. Only John and the women who had supported Jesus stood by at the cross, willing and able to risk everything to be with him. Few of us suffer such desertion. Most of the friends who hurt us are more weak than traitorous. Still all the disappointments that we suffer can teach us a greater truth.

Only God is unfailing, and even with God we've got to get our criteria straight. God is not bound to support us on the terms that we expect or want. We have to write God a blank check, if we are to find divine providence completely satisfactory. We cannot write other human beings such a check (though we approach doing so when we fall head over heels in love), because we know that they are limited, weak, sinful, ignorant, and all the other ungodly things that we ourselves are.

What the terminally ill most need from their friends is prayer, the token and substance of support at the deepest level, where we all face the abysmal mystery of God. I use the word "abysmal" advisedly, without negative overtones, focusing on the fathomless, unsoundable quality of the divine being. It is a "terrible" thing to fall into the hands of the living God, as scripture says, because the living God scarily measures all of us and can be measured by none. We are out of our depth, our league, our minds when we deal with the living God. We are in over our heads, even over our hearts. Should our hearts condemn us, as they are bound to if we are honest, God is greater. Should our folly whisper that we have it made with God, are righteous, God is again greater, taking away any guarantees.

Our best friends realize that terminal illness makes this theology pressing. No longer is it merely bookish teaching, sayings that entice the mind but require no action. Now, we have to repent of everything that we used to do to keep the incomprehensibility of God at arms' length. Now, these are home truths, ideally become the measures for our soul.

Plato spoke of the unseen measure. Christians ought to speak of a measure unmeasured and unmeasurable, as well as unseen. Nothing comes before God, is a more primary reference. Prayer expresses an intuition of this singularly crucial truth, and prayer is where we are most likely to have such a truth imprinted on our soul.

The God we meet in prayer, if we manufacture even a smidgin of faithfulness, is too much for us—a cloud for our minds, a dark night for our factoidal spirits. This is the real God, whose most sacramental countenance is the scandalous Christ. A stumbling block to the Jew in us, and to the Gentile in us foolishness, this eschatological man of God brings all the truly faithful to their knees. In the prayer through which they gather up all whom their hearts caress, Christ brings before God all their friends. So the people who pray for us out of their depths are our greatest benefactors. By their prayer, we can know our real friends.

31. *Feeling Better*

One of the changes accompanying my improved condition has been a quieting of my sense of urgency. I have resumed the assumption of the healthy that they have time to negotiate with the world, to think about basic matters objectively, in detachment. This change involves certain obvious advantages and disadvantages. It helps me to possess my spirit in peace and patience, moving it gently to the issues of death and divine providence. But it also puts me in danger of forgetting that pain and death are not long ago and far away, or of forgetting that multiple myeloma is an incurable, terminal cancer.

Even when sickest, I never thought that my death was imminent. Slowly, since the diagnosis of my cancer, I have appropriated the thought that I am likely to die younger than the normal lifespan for white American males. In some ways death has become more familiar, a regular at my bar and grill, as has the comforting thought that we all die, sooner or later. My cancer is not disgracefully singular. All death can seem disgraceful, even obscene, inasmuch as we associate goodness and God with wholeness and life. But no death need go unredeemed, inasmuch as we associate the resurrection of Jesus with the death he accepted freely, for us and our salvation.

Sometimes I think profitably about the amazing advantages of having a God who has known our human condition down to its marrow and suffered our mortality. How God, the deathless source of all life, can have died escapes human understanding, but there it is, plain as the traditional Creed. The one who holds the act of existence in Jesus, who for our sakes "came down from heaven," and "suffered, died, and was buried," was divine, the Son of God living in the bosom of the Father, God from God, Light from Light.

Traditional Christian theology speaks of a "communication of idioms," such that we can predicate human attributes of the Son, and divine attributes of Jesus, because of the union of divine and human natures in him. He is one person. The same person who lives with the Father and Spirit was born of Mary and died on Calvary. This can be interpreted so as to minimize his humanity, but it should not be. It also can be interpreted so as to lessen the scandal of saying that God died on the cross, but it should not be, least of all by people with a terminal illness.

To say that God died on the cross is not to say, of course, that this death annihilated God or extinguished the divine awareness. It is only to say that the Word Incarnate experienced fully the end of ordinary human existence that death denotes. In dying Jesus ceased to be what he had been when living, just as all the rest of us cease to be what we were. He has preceded me in giving up his spirit. I cannot understand what his resurrection entailed, except that it suggests a new mode of being human. In that new mode, death must appear differently than it does to the unresurrected. To the unresurrected, death is a frightening terminus. To the resurrected, death must appear as a blessed transition, the passage they had to make to their new, more desirable status.

In moments of calm, induced by good health and considerable pondering of what the terminal in "terminal illness" may imply, I find myself thinking well of death. I have stopped thinking about pain, perhaps foolishly, to concentrate on the positive connotations of finishing—coming to term. If our lives were endless, what would be their drama? If we were always to be seeking, wanting, never finding, how would we avoid frustration?

32. My God

The God who has beckoned to me during the past year, whom I have most probed in the dead of night, the cold of what Ingmar Bergman called "the hour of the wolf," is more ontological than psychological, more medieval than modern. This God, no Jungian archetype, is more real than my feelings, more stable than my moods, the depth and constitution of whatever is, the most basic fact of my facticity.

If I am, if I really exist and am not a dream, then I rest in God. Nothing can be without God, and the being of any thing belongs to God. My being does not come from me. I can no more give myself being than I can give myself life. My being comes from God, who provides the reality of my reality, the isness of my isness. God is the act speaking me into my act of existing here, now, historically—as a person composing a story willy-nilly.

To contact God, deal with God, connect myself to the divine purpose, I need only appreciate my existence. Let me merely sink to the roots of my self and I find a dark, impenetrable ground I can responsibly call God. Let me simply follow the outreach of my mind or heart, press beyond the sensate world around me in search of an invisible perfection, and I can reasonably think that I am projecting myself toward God, by God's support, lure, call. There is no I without God, no humanity, no world. Everything that makes a human being is derived from, is connected to, an immensity, an infinity, an absoluteness toward which we point with the small word, "God."

The treasure is not the word itself (though we will not despise the word, if we are wise) but the reality to which the word points, inevitably falteringly. The point is not what the concept expressed in the word can denote but what the action, the drive of the mind and heart, generating the concept reaches toward. We would not seek God if we were not human—incarnate beings defined by something, someone, without limits. We cannot be human without God, and the history of our worst inhumanities is the story of how we have tried to play God, or to do without God—have refused to keep stretching toward the indefinable, and so given up, reneged, on our constitutional charge to become holy.

Jesus stands in the center of this mystery as the incarnation of the indefinable. He was credible during his life because of the power of his goodness, which could heal the sick and raise the dead. He remains credible after his death because he did not end, because the Father raised him and so defeated death. For people with terminal illness, with a heavy message from death announcing its arrival in the near future, Jesus makes the being of God in our being, the nearness of God in our spirits, close and specific.

Can it be that the being that makes us stand out from nothingness both utters itself eternally and compacts that utterance into flesh? Can we responsibly believe that the story of the resurrection of Jesus ratifies the claim that in him God gave a terminal word, worked a definitive revelation, that orients even the stars and the seas? The more fully we experience the abysmal depths on which we float, the more unlikely yet wonderfully fitting the Christian mysteries become. Jesus was so good, so powerful, so innocent and resurrectible because, as chapter one of Colossians sings lovingly, "in him all things hold together."

33. Measuring the Immeasurable

The Word of God is unlimited. It exists at another level, in another order, from that which we enter when we try to imagine the reaches of the galaxies, the time or extent of the Big Bang. We measure some of these natural things, using reason to make sense of infinity, but we ourselves are not the measure. All our final measuring is negative. The best we can do with ultimacy is to imagine no bounds, no hindrances, no death. If we are the measure, the world is mortal and joy does not reign. We die and there is no hope for happiness. But if Jesus, one of us without limit, can be our measure, then humanity is more than death and suffering, humanity can be the primal sacrament of God.

Few of my friends, even my academic friends, seem to wonder consistently how to integrate an ontological understanding of God with the sacramentality of Jesus. If the surest way to think that God is with me, supporting me in my great need, is to discover God to be the foundation and marrow of my being, why should I deal with a finite, crucified enfleshment of my God—a folly to the reasoning mind and a scandal to the believing heart?

Can it be that what I hear in the story of Christ, is the key to how the being of God works in my being? Can the death now developing mindlessly in my bone marrow be held, limited, contained by the utterance of

God that proved stronger than the cross of Calvary?

I must cling to Jesus, died and risen, if my sense of the God holding me in being is to save me. Clinging to Jesus, I open myself to the Father and the Spirit, through whom Jesus defined himself. This definition was active—lived rather than speculated, performed more than pondered. For Jesus it was connatural, spontaneous. For me it is more labored, obscure. The reality is the same in both cases. What Jesus believed operates in my depths and provides my surest definition, if I am truly a Christian, someone inserted into the mystery of Jesus that Christians call reality and salvation.

The divinity that comes alive in the names Father, Son, and Spirit is the wellspring of my being. It shares its eternal circulations of light and life and love with me even as it creates me, keeps me in existence, and empowers me to act (even to act against it).

There is no opposition between Jesus and the Trinity. The Trinity expresses both what Jesus felt he was involved with when he prayed and what we find we are involved with when we let Jesus take us to the depths of ourselves, to the fullest outreach of our minds and hearts, to the strongest remedies for our world's evils.

34. Curing and Healing

Some native American tribes have used "medicine" to summarize their sense of what gives power, health, vitality, healing. People concerned with healing, perhaps in contrast to curing, tend to widen their sense of health care. Healing involves the mind and heart, the spirit as well as the body. People cured of cancer in the sense of enjoying a full remission of the disease would not be healed if great fear of cancer or unhappiness about life in general still oppressed them. In reflecting on what terminal illness has made of medicine—our hospitals and clinics, doctors and nurses—I find I am more interested in healing than curing.

I have great reason to thank the medical establishment. Left untreated, my multiple myeloma probably would have killed me in six months. The statistics still are not encouraging, but since spending a month in the hospital about a year ago, I have had more good days than bad. Indeed, all my days, both those filled with pain and those blessed with peace, have been a wonder. The days when I have had to take drugs have whispered one set of lessons, while the days when I have felt fairly normal have whispered another. "Number my days," I have prayed from time to time. "Compose this time into something beautiful."

We have medicine and need hospitals because to be human is to be liable to sickness or wounding. Things can go wrong with our bodies, as with our emotions and spirits. Sometimes experts can make such things right again, or at least can lessen their wrongness. If we call "pain" the immediate, visceral effect of wrongness, the unavoidable sign that something is out of joint, we can distinguish pain from "suffering," calling the latter the full, psychosomatic experience of pain. Then we can try to endure it, make sense of it, rearrange our life so as to deal with it.

Medicine concerns itself with both pain and suffering, unless it is hopelessly mechanistic. None of the hospitals or clinics that I have visited was hopelessly mechanistic. The vast majority of the doctors and nurses who have treated me have tried to ameliorate my suffering as well as my pain.

From the experience of support groups organized for people suffering from particular illnesses, we know that healing can come from a variety of sources. Doctors and nurses can provide considerable healing, whether or not they themselves have been seriously ill. So can fellow patients, ordinary people who are not ill, and individual patients themselves. Healing runs a range, implies a gamut, that roots it in our common, bedrock human condition. None of us goes through life without suffering. All of us are afflicted by physical or emotional or spiritual pain. When we find ourselves hurting we are simply actualizing a constant human potential. No man or woman walking the earth is invulnerable. Every one of us needs help, at least from time to time.

I find just thinking thoughts such as these helpful, healing. I find minimizing the singularity of my terminal illness beneficial in itself. If you do not have cancer, you have some other pain or worry. If today is completely sunny for you, tomorrow may well not be. I do not mean to cast human existence under a cloud, throw forth a great wet blanket. But I do mean to lay out, expose, the vulnerability and mortality built into the human condition, and to draw a proper comfort from it.

If I am singular, idiosyncratic, I stand apart from the mainstream of human beings, outside the human community. But if my cancer is neither unusual nor the most significant thing about me, I find my fear of it lessened. A mechanism in my bone marrow has gone awry, for reasons presently unknown. In your case, a mechanism in the stock market may have gone awry, for reasons known or unknown, and you too have something to fear, to bring back under emotional control. Cancer threatens me with ruin of one sort. The collapse of your bank account threatens you with ruin of another sort. We both have a problem, a lot of work to do. You may be glad that you do not have my problem, that your problem is only money. But I may see that solving my problem will teach me things well beyond the stock market, things you have yet to imagine. In some cases, though, no time of suffering need be lost. In both cases God is sure to have lessons for us.

35. Reforming the Church

It is easy to criticize the church and terribly hard to reform it. We Christians are the church, all of us believers, and we are a stiff-necked people. Divided for centuries, we have come to love our divisions, thinking them necessary to our sense of ourselves. Who would we be, if we were not different from Baptists or Orthodox, if they were more like us than different? How would we remain the apple of God's eye if Buddhists and Muslims could be saved? The ecumenical movement stalled when church leaders realized what consummating it would ask of them, but this stalling struck many a responsive chord in the pews of the different denominations.

So, now, we have to ask again what it means to call ourselves "the people of God," what reforms that image imposes. The church is always to be reformed, if Protestant theology is perceptive. The holiness of the church comes only from God—all human ordinances are imperfect. I have been most saddened by the unwillingness of church leaders to cash out the central theology of Christian faith so as to maximize the freedom of their people.

The central theology of Christian faith includes the confession that we cannot know what God is, and that whatever we say about God, God is always more unlike than like our saying. Handing on these traditional theses, church leaders find themselves at a crossroads. They can interpret the theses as a writ of intellectual freedom, as well as an encouragement of an Augustinian ethic rooted in "love and do what you will." Or they can interpret them to justify extreme caution, as though God were a great darkness and only they held the pencil-flash of light.

The Spirit of God is the only instructor adequate for the entirety of our journey. The Spirit of God knows each of us through and through, as no body of ecclesiastical legislators can. Yes, the Spirit of God loves concord, does not raise up prideful rebels. But the Spirit of God also loves excellence, has no envy of wit or energy. The Spirit of God is erotic, passionate for God, and for all who love God spiritedly. The Spirit of God is no puritan, no petty lawyer, no hack. Would that the Spirit were more manifest in the Christian churches.

The church is healthiest when most aware of the primacy of the Spirit. It is most encouraging when it tells its children to trust their instincts, confess their sins, and renew their love of the game. A church that is not playful, does not love the game and play it well, is much less than what we require, if we are to make the church our first community. Not alert and playful, it is not the communion of saints, the body of Christ, the eschatological community of salvation. It is not the great sign lifted up on the hill, the desire of all the nations. It is all too human, all too readily dismissed.

Not being any of these good things as well as we ought, as fully as we might, we, the church, show ourselves to be deeply sinful. At the least, we are not God, and we can only speak for God modestly. We have little right to hurl anathemas, much reason to ask the world to forgive us. The charge laid on us nowadays, when so much of the world does not love us, is to love the world, the creation of God, selflessly, seeking no temporal gain, no spiritual advantage, that would taint the memory of Christ.

I want to die as a child of the church, and I know that only I myself can prevent this. I want to keep the faith so long handed down, so beautiful to the great cloud of witnesses. The church has been my home, spiritually more than politically or physically. Much as I've despised churchiness, Uriah Heep in cassock or preacher's gown, I've learned to pray, and love, and laugh in the church, and so to sense what a healthy view of death requires. For all these reasons, when I pray for the church I first say, "Deo gratias": "Thanks be to God."

36. The Power of Creative Thinking

The thinking that makes me more realistic about both my situation and my faith is a large part of the "work" that my spirit asks of me. Indeed, I believe that all our spirits ask something like this of us. This is the main reason that I chose to work first as a teacher and then as a writer. I think that our most human, intimate obligation is to gain the understanding of our condition necessary to live wisely. In this context, death obviously can be a boon. The many religious schools that counsel meditating on death know what they are doing. From *The Tibetan Book of the Dead* to *The Imitation of Christ*, many of the most stimulating treatments of wisdom make meditation on death central.

Apart from this inner-directed work, oriented to gaining the perspective necessary to handle terminal illness with some grace, I have had to ponder my outer, professional work as a practiced writer. For sixteen years, I have concentrated on writing, with my wife producing more than seventy books. Now, with time short, on what ought I to spend my writing time? Two possibilities have stretched before me, one stemming from what I am most drawn to write, the other stemming from what outsiders most need to know. At the moment, the first possibility seems the more compelling.

In the past, Denise and I have written numerous textbooks, under the conviction that serving college students palatable meals of religious wisdom is a good work, and one somewhat neglected, somewhat despised, by the academic mandarins. Now, however, I feel that we have discharged our debts to students and ought to move as a new spirit pushes us.

This is a goal for which we had long been working, but only by shifting my orientation have I actually moved onto a new track and brought our goal closer to realization. One specific project that has come to represent this new orientation is a novel, *The Year of the Bad,* that I have pledged myself to begin. It may turn out to be one of the world's worst novels (remember, though, how Andrew Greeley's pulps sell), but I anticipate doing it with relish, wasting time properly.

The Year of the Bad beckons as an opportunity to reflect, reminisce, and imagine things too real actually to have happen. Such things live in the realm of what might have been, where the real estate costs are prohibitive. The realm of what might have been, the scholastic theologians' "futuribles," is a subsection of the mind of God. In the mind of God occurs everything that might have been, as well as all that has been, is, or will be. The mind of God is exhaustive, a warehouse like the alaya-vijnana, the "storehouse consciousness" that fascinates Yogacara Buddhists. Just as the law of nature is merely a subset of the eternal law of creation housed in the divine mind, so the realms that authors wander, poets conjure up, musicians and scientists visit—all the permutations of human fantasy—sport, cavort there. When we imagine seriously, responsibly, though ideally playfully as well, we take ourselves to the mind of God, God's are the galleries we pace.

I'm interested in the relations that might have been, had I chosen differently at critical junctures, or stumbled into parenthood, or set up as a counselor, or taken multiple myeloma more, or less, seriously. I'm even more interested in making people, creating characters, describing places I've never been, encounters that never happened.

One of the large zones that "God" would cover, were our spiritualities more properly negative, is all this otherworldliness, all these universes to which no one has ever traveled in body. I am not moving into science fiction. I am not expecting to make people, create characters, tell stories especially well. I am only expecting to make "retirement" real, the sabbath actual, by deliberating "wasting" time on non-profit activities, occupations undertaken only for their own sakes.

If leisure is the basis of culture, and cultus is close to play, then retirement may become a time of deeper culture and better worship. That is my hope. As I think about what I want to do, as a means of achieving what I want to become, things that are free, uncommercial, done with amateur purity come to mind. I want to visit the places that memory now catalogues as crucial, talk again with the people who most shaped my soul. I want to stop caring about the index of literacy, all the tests of textbook publishers that report how few words today's students understand.

The birds sing because they must, unto the glory of their creator. The best poets write because they must, if their lives are to remain worth living. Religious people pray dutifully, but if they hear the Way in the morning, in the evening they can die content. In retirement they are instinctively Taoist, even the most Confucian among them.

37. Word and Sacrament

In the months ahead, I hope to write about the gospel of John. This gospel cries out for a lectio divina, a reading concerned mainly with spiritual sense. It is the most intriguing of the gospels, the one where the Christology is the highest (the divinity of Jesus is the clearest). It is also the most sacramental, seeing signs and wonders everywhere.

For decades this namesake evangelist has been my favorite, not the least because of his irony. His Jesus does not suffer fools gladly, and his man-born-blind gives the pharisaic mind exactly what it deserves (see John 9:1–41). What is the implication of this irony in the middle of revelation? What sting ought the back-of-the-hand of the man-born-blind to carry? Why should we, and should we not, identify the pharisaic mind with church bureaucrats of all ages? How does it happen that the most incarnational gospel is the most mystical?

These are only some of the questions, a bit of the intrigue, that working leisurely, for the joy of it, on the gospel of John brings to mind. When I move from my favorite scripture to my favorite sacrament, the eucharist begets similar questions, an analogous intrigue. John tells me that "in him [Jesus] was life." The eucharist is the bread of life, the medicine of immortality, precisely the antidote to terminal illness that people of faith long to find.

Flatfooted interpreters think that only males can preside at the eucharist, because the president must physically resemble Jesus, the main actor. Richer interpreters intuit that much more than a passion play is at stake. Principally, Jesus, the Johannine "bread of life," works with the Jewish seder to create a meal through which he may commune with his followers, and they with one another, at the depths of life and death. Certainly, his sacrifice on the cross casts a shadow, riveting the passover, the exodus from Egypt, onto the issue of bedrock human mortality. Even more central is Jesus' memorial of the love of God that has sought, in a dozen ways, to take flesh and dwell among us, to draw near and take us into the divine relations, which, we recall in passing, are deathless.

When you have celebrated the eucharist, enacted Jesus' meal, day after day for decades, the coin of bread and wine, listening and consuming, becomes the standard in your personal economy. You pray to the Father, standing where Jesus does, and you imagine the encircling movement of the Spirit, the love proceeding from the Father. You eat so that your life may be taken over, since you know that what you eat, whose flesh you consume, is stronger than you and deathless. You drink recalling the blood poured out for the many, but recalling the wine of gladness even more. A messianic banquet comes to mind, a great party in the hall of heaven, to model your feasting upon. You think of the daily bread for which the prayer of Jesus asks, all the provisions that God alone can supply.

Sometimes the symbolism seems endless, because the images are so basic. We live and die, eat and drink, and always we yearn for love. We choose words that we call canonical, events that we believe are paradigmatic, summoning them into the present. In the measure that our imaginations are Christian, the paradigms of Jesus become privileged, and no event is more paradigmatic than his death and resurrection, his paschal movement from Good Friday to Easter Sunday.

These are images, actions, privileged words by which I have lived for nearly fifty years, so it seems a homecoming to write about them. I am eager to think deeply and lovingly about all that they can be when we let them ring in our inner ear, let them touch our hearts and stir our affections.

Books on the eucharist and the gospel of John spring from my priestly imagination, which has remained strong, despite the desire of church officials that I not exercise it. They did not see how it could be compatible with marriage. They did not see that the genius of Christianity is its sacramentality, which flows directly from the Incarnation.

Food and sex, like words and actions, require a love of matter, if they are to prosper, seem good in the eyes of heaven. Average church leaders, pharisees, do not love matter, have no soul erotic for precisely human beauty. They live by prudence, caution, fear rather than joy, love, or creativity. Life is hard enough, without the burden of their lack of humor. Sacraments thin to bareness and bone, if left in their papery hands. As I have

— 96 —

thought sabbatically, in the free zone that the Letter to the Hebrews associates with the divine rest, I have reclaimed the priestly from the clerical. Along the way, I reasserted the rights of all believers to the beauty of God's Word and Sacrament.

I shall attempt these books, as I shall attempt a novel, with humor and hope for mischief. One of the delights one can find occasionally in the alcoves where cancer patients receive chemotherapy is rebels dancing on the devil's grave. Peasant, earthy, a kind of pissing away one's fears, this cast of mind may become exactly Christian, just the thing that the man-born-mortal needs when the pharisees of his time, obtuse as ever, forget that no cleric fails to die, and all bodies have to deal with food, sex, and songs for soulful singing.

38. Changing My World View

How has moving into the half-life of partial remission of cancer, the funny hut mid-way along the mountain trail, affected my perception of world events? How it ought to affect them? These are the questions now on the table.

I have become inured to the follies of the nations—Iraq, the former Yugoslavia, my own country. Similarly, I have become inured to the stupidities of commercial television. But the shock I felt while watching news of the world when my diagnosis was new has remained with me. Why do the nations rage? Why does a popular culture care what a rock star wears, how high a basketball superstar can jump?

Life seen to be passing should be life held to be precious. The nations who go to war so easily, the monomanical dictators who make the gutters run with blood, either think they are immortal, exceptions to biology's first rule, or they think that all human existence is meaningless, with no judgment of God restoring either meaning or life. The plainest facts of human experience do not register on such people, make no impact, largely because no Christian faith gives death a context, shows how it need not destroy our dignity.

Recently we visited Graz, Austria, and found ourselves only an hour from the fighting among Serbs, Croats, and Bosnian Muslims in the former Yugoslavia. We listened to representatives of these three groups interpret the past five hundred years of their history and fashion apologias for their current barbarism. Looking inside, I found myself following the disgust of my spirit like a chain down to an anchor on the ocean floor. Death was the anchor, the bite into reality that made the chain hold.

The people speaking to us of past history and interpreting current events had to be well aware of death. They also had to be well aware of outrages outstripping death in evil, such as the systematic rape of 60,000 Bosnian Muslim women in an effort to destroy the Bosnian bloodline—an effort at genocide. However, neither in what they said as spokesmen for their ethnic group, nor in what they intimated of their personal outlook, did any of these representatives show that death had led him to abandon history to God, or to pray for God's mercy on both his own benighted people and the enemies they have hated so long.

I was trying to listen sympathetically, ignoring the pain in my weakened back. I was trying to humble my American spirit, telling it that I would never understand people formed by centuries of ethnic violence. But I was not succeeding, because the pain in my back, the knowledge in my psyche, was making me call all the parties to the bloodshed stupid—criminally, sinfully stupid. How could they not have eyes to see that the survival of their children was incalculably more important than their wounded pride, or their memory of past atrocities, or their lust for land, or whatever other disordered passions possessed them? How long would it be before the stench in their souls rose up to their noses and, like strong smelling salts, cleared the fog from their brains? I wished that at least one of the panelists had been a woman, because I have found women more likely than men to retain a clear brain about war. Certainly, women can have long memories, but more often than not their love of their children, their visceral, uterine ties to life, keep them from the madness of male bloodlust, the folly of men hell-bent on revenge.

I never got as close to the events in Somalia, the efforts of the United Nations to keep the local warlords from stealing the grain standing between the common people and starvation. On another front, the feckless pursuit of peace in the Middle East, between Arabs and Israelis, has ceased to interest me, because there are few heroes for whom to root, few people of wisdom saying or doing what obviously must be said and done. There can be no peace in the Middle East, as there can be no routing of starvation in Somalia, until the common good comes to prevail over individual advantage, until all parties repent of their own sins and forgive the sins of others. All the rest is rhetoric, as useless as it is easy. Certainly, repentance and forgiveness write a tall order. Nonetheless, a strong sense of death, a keen awareness of death's hands on the throats of one's children, could whittle it down overnight. With all the blood shed since 1948, why do neither Jews nor Arabs really want peace? Why do both remain so stupid?

What do a few kilometers of dusty turf matter, when none of us has surety of the morrow? How can it be difficult to go halfway, hoist three-fifths of the common burden, when the gain is life and the loss is ruin? You will say that people not galvanized by their mortality are unlikely to see things this clearly, and you will be right. But I must say in return that nothing is more obvious than our mortality. In the world's trouble spots, the bodies pile up like sandbags along a dike. And so what you say and what I say begin to converge, despite our different starting points. What we converge upon is the mystery of human folly, which is also the mystery of human sin.

39. The Eve of Destruction

Looking at the grotesquerie parading through world events, I find it hard not to despair of our species. At the least, one has to conclude that we human beings seem incapable of gaining the wisdom or showing the good judgment necessary for our survival. The starvation shaming Somalia stems from folly, as does the enmity shaming the Middle East. The catastrophe building in the degradation of the earth's ecosystems reveals an even greater folly, because the solutions are more obvious and the stakes considerably higher.

Who has breathed the air of Los Angeles or Tokyo or Mexico City and not intuited that our modern, industrialized way of life has no long-term future? Who has looked hard at the housing in any of these cities and not sensed that contemporary history has taken a horribly wrong turn? Despite these commonplace observations, we seem incapable of shutting the engines down, turning the ship around. We know the direction of safety, what we must do to reach solid ground, but we cannot or will not muster the political will required.

Are we in fact too flawed to avoid destruction? Is our fault, the crack in our being, so wide and deep that we are doomed? No one can answer questions such as these, but if we make death our interpretational lens, human folly seems all the greater: How much plainer could the lesson be? If we will not listen to Moses, not even one returning from the dead could instruct us.

Most of what people cling to, of what keeps them from reason and reform, are baubles and bagatelles. Like John of the Cross's tiny cord that holds the sparrow, keeping it from flying free in the heavens, our attachments tend to be ludicrous. We won't reform our systems of transportation, because we have to have private cars. We won't give up beef in our diet, because we love McDonalds. We think we need hundreds of chemically-based consumer products, the majority of which are trash. We won't reform the banking and trade that have become part and parcel of our ecological dysfunction, because we let lobbyists rule our parliaments. And, most challenging to me, we won't generate the new religious visions, the new loves for creation, that could blast our self-centeredness away.

All these things we could do, if we hungered for peace and justice, hurt to our souls at nature's ruin. All these things we could do, if we made death our tutor in the beauty of life, the wonder of life, the preciousness of our planet. Who will save us from our bone-deep ignorance, redeem us from our dim-witted selves? These are not new questions. From the beginning of time people have raised them, especially people carried to mountain crags by death.

The best result of remembering death is a renewed love of life. Those in whom the Spirit of God moves most clearly are those who love children most dearly, hate war most passionately. The knock of death at the door ought to make my faith more fully sacramental, incarnational, grateful to the God who said let there be light, life, love. Certainly, terminal illness also ought to detach me from false treasures, baubles, and bagatelles. But after an initial severance from ephemeral things, I ought to return to the world for which Jesus died, overcome my disgust, and foster my love.

World events arrange themselves best when the love of God that took Jesus to the cross and raised him from the grave has decided the place settings. The messianic banquet comes into clearest focus when goodness, rather than worldly power, determines who sits closest to the lord. The beatitudes of Jesus scramble the judgments that dominate our newspapers. The Sermon on the Mount goes unheeded in Washington, London, and Tokyo. Wisdom cries out from mismatch between plenty and poverty. Death itself seems to weep, ashamed that so few hear it.

Terminal illness has not made me wise, but it has made me sober. Often I find myself watching Jesus weep over Jerusalem. Generation after generation, we repeat the same follies. We think that being depends on having. We think that the real is the most passionately felt. Above all, we deny the brutal, freeing fact of death. We will not quiet our souls, listen from the heart, simplify our selves so that we want only what may be stronger. Love is strong as death, perhaps even stronger. Grace abounds over sin, if we know where to go. I should know these things, for my education has been privileged. I forget these things, time after time, so I have no platform for preaching.

Unable now to do very much, ending without much money or power, I find myself a desert father. Whispering late at night, he says that I will love the world best, best discharge the chores of membership in the human community, by praying for all the world's suffering, that multitude that none can count. This is something I can do, and so something that I must. All the rest is commentary. The center is a silent plea.

40. Looking at the Church

How does the church look "under the aspect of eternity," with death shaping one's horizon? In my case, the church looks like an institution for which I should be more grateful than often I've been, although it is also a serious disappointment.

There are no theologians to speak of, no poets of God, apart from religious communities. In the Christian case, my case, the religious community that has nourished the people who have most helped my faith is the church. Though my formation was Roman Catholic, I have followed the general drift of liberal, educated Christians into an ecumenical understanding and love of the church, taking my Christian nourishment wherever it has seemed palatable. For an understanding of death, the medieval mystics have been helpful, as has the theology of the twentieth-century Jesuit, Karl Rahner, which makes God our absolute future.

Working with the mainstream of Christian tradition, steeping himself in the Church Fathers and Thomas Aquinas, Rahner reconceived human nature as an outreach for God. Everywhere, human beings are seeking God, who is the horizon of our knowing, the global context and term of our desiring and loving. Everywhere, God offers the divine being, makes the divine life present, to encourage a salvific knowing and sustain a desire and love for heaven. God pours out grace everywhere. We cannot enter any realm, physical or spiritual, where God has not preceded us. We cannot be, exist, without God's grant. God gives us our human definition.

The implications of this view of both human nature and the Christian God are enormous. One of the most pertinent ramifications for people with terminal illness is the conception of God as our absolute future.

"Absolute" means "unconditioned." There are no qualifications to the primacy, the sufficiency, of God. There is nothing on which God depends. To make "absolute" an adjective modifying "future" is to take away any implicit restrictions. When conjoined with God, "future" opens out endlessly. God is where we are all heading, "the beckoning whither of our now." God is where we want to go, are designed to go, in many ways go willy-nilly. Pascal said that we would not seek God, had we not already found God. We do find God. God is ready to hand, when we interpret the future absolutely.

Now, death is my future, and your future as well. Death therefore correlates with God, though precisely how no one can tell us. We can tell ourselves, though, that we have been made for God. Our hearts are restless until they rest in God. Yes, they can rest in God now, in time, while we live here, in this world that God has created. But that rest is fragile, vulnerable, imperiled. Apart from a mystical action of God that binds us to the divine being inescapably, we have to soldier along, comporting ourselves like pilgrims. As we do this, hoping that God shares our journey, we can realize that the absoluteness of God makes all our failures, and all our successes, provisional. It is well for us to move through the stations of life gracefully, but only reaching our end will complete us.

The church has offered me many other truths by which to set my course, compose my soul. As I try to wrap up my intellectual affairs I draw upon them. The secular world is not a rich resource, does not have much to offer, when it comes to dealing with death. The secular world runs from death, distracts itself from death, in good part because death makes so many secular concerns seem shallow. The church says that death is not the end, though in faith we should call it a hiatus. The church says that we do not transmigrate smoothly, coming back in another capsule for another ride. Neither do we cease to be, or start to be only as disembodied spirits.

At the moment of death, in the twinkling of an eye, we are changed. We finally get the chance to sum ourselves up, say yes or no to the lives we've made and been given. For the first time, we can accept or reject fully the selves we've become. If either our acceptance or our rejection makes God our absolute future, the great love of our lives, we can hope to have passed judgment. We cannot imagine how judgment will occur, or what its aftermath will be, but we can intuit that gaining or losing full intimacy with God will be the crux of the outcome.

For these and a great number of other good thoughts and helpful images, I bless the church. On the other hand, appropriating a medical death sentence has also increased my frustration with the church, my sadness at its failures. It is not the place of freedom and joy that it might be, were God its absolute future. Regularly it is petty, legalistic, practically faithless. The institutional church seeks its own advantage far more than its master did. Its leaders want more of the world's pleasures, goods, honors. Nowadays they do not welcome the best and the brightest, because these are bound to be critical.

Moreover, the church nurtures a bias against women, refusing to break with its historic patriarchy. Often it is obsessive about sex, to the great diminishment of its people's joy. Often it forgets that its only function is service, since its master came not to be ministered unto but to minister to others. Girding its loins, a more faithful church would kneel each day to wash the feet of the poor. It would not restrict this symbolism or substance to Holy Thursday. It would be canonical for both Lent and ordinary time.

41. Healing and the Mind

It is a great gift from medical science to be cured of one's disease. Certainly, if offered a cure for my multiple myeloma I would not hesitate to take it. But whether or not I am cured, I can make progress toward a significant healing, perhaps one day reaching the point where I can say that I feel quite whole and blessed.

I love to contemplate a medical practice that aims at this kind of healing. I find it wonderful news that in many parts of the United States, a quest for wholeness shapes the practice of many hospitals and retreat houses. The hospice movement is a great ray of light. Places for healing-retreats embody a philosophy of medicine both sound and deep. Beyond the borders of medicine and psychology or medicine and religion that a narrow chart-maker might draw, many people are seeking ways to heal the entire human person, body and soul, private and social.

The people who impress me the most are those who adopt a holistic view of healing while respecting the gains that medical science has made and the technological helps it can offer. They do not despise chemotherapy or surgery, any more than they despise diet, exercise, meditation, or patients' sharing their experiences in groups. The healers most attractive to me are open, not dogmatic. They are also critical, slow to embrace any fads or simplistic panaceas. They value medical science for the precision and testing that it favors. At the same time, they recognize the apparent fact that more than physical, measurable factors are at work in all serious illnesses.

Whether such factors as a patient's emotional state, his or her sense of loneliness or social support, produce physical changes (for example, in the immune system) is a matter of considerable medical interest. We need not wait for confirmation in terms of chemical studies, however, to open ourselves to the commonsensical position that social or psychological factors influence a patient's will to live, and that a patient's will to live can be as significant as the results of his or her CAT scan or blood work.

I find myself imagining a future medical practice that will put itself in a fail-safe, win-win situation. By continuing to develop its scientific understanding of disease, and a correlative medical technology, it will continue to cure physical disorders—aberrant mechanisms in bones and blood, pathological organs. By associating these attacks on disease with efforts to lessen patients' illnesses, improve their experience of being sick, and ameliorate their suffering, this ideal future medical practice will improve the healing it can provide, helping people regain as much all-around health and many-dimensional wholeness as possible. Finally, by dealing with the ultimate issues of meaning, the full import of death and life, this future medical practice might both lessen patients' anxieties and enrich the experience, professional and personal, of medical practitioners.

This presumes, of course, that both patients and physicians are beings simultaneously physical, psychological, and spiritual. It is to say that healing and wholeness connote bodily, emotional, and metaphysical or religious factors. In any final, adequate analysis, we cannot separate the pathogenic cells, the feelings of fear and loneliness, and the questions about what happens at death and what we should stress as life-time grows short.

It is not fair to ask any single person to be expert in all these matters, but it is fair to ask all parties to the creation of our future medical procedures to give all these matters their due. Moreover, it is more than fair to insist that medicine, like education and the other central institutional forces in our culture, understand itself, present itself, and function as a fully humane enterprise.

All the people involved with medicine are simply people. None of them has ever seen God or been mistaken by the sane for God. Each is mortal. Each is vulnerable to cancer, depression, and wonder about ultimate meanings, doubts about how to live. The more successfully we turn this common, radically equalizing humanity into patience, sympathy, and properly leisurely treatment of whole people, the better we shall realize the marvelous potential in human medicine. The less we submit to simplistic options for either technological improvements or support groups, the more adequately we shall envision and imagine human healing. Terminal illness helps to clarify all this, because terminal illness so obviously is simultaneously physical, emotional, and metaphysical. Whatever patients with terminal illnesses can do to make their experience bear on the future orientation of health care will lessen the waste that their sufferings threaten.

42. Education in Ultimate Perspective

How does higher education look when one is meditating about death? How successfully does it pass scrutiny? I have spent over thirty-five years in higher education, so the pros and cons are familiar. Nonetheless, I have been surprised at the thinness, the superficiality, in current American higher education that my terminal illness has provoked me to find. In the past year, the irrelevance of most academic discourse has become oppressive.

I believe in knowledge for its own sake. I do not think that praxis, let alone ideology, should rule what scholars study or how intellectuals should think. I do think, however, that reality should be our great passion. Relatedly, I think that "reality" is not so variable, multi-cultural, or phantom a notion as many academicians seem to think. Nature sets many of the parameters for a realistic assessment of where we are placed and what factors affect the world around us. Although nature is mysterious, boxes within boxes, it is also sufficiently objective to furnish us rights and wrongs.

Cancer may be a pluralistic disease, a family of diseases, but each member of the family appears in cellular disorders that are susceptible to physical treatment. Such treatment (chemotherapy, for example), may or may not cure the cancer in question, but medical scientists can measure the effects of the treatment and determine whether the tumors have or have not shrunk.

Human nature is more plastic than physical nature, but it is not completely protean. All human beings die. All are ignorant, in the sense that none knows all there is to know. Indeed, none knows, empirically, the answers to the simple but crucial questions of where we came from and where we are going. History, along with an examination of conscience, tells us that human beings are also morally imperfect. Beyond the fact that we die and do not know everything, we are not as good, as honest and loving, as the part of us called "conscience" says we should be.

Just as the natural sciences are not realistic unless they admit the data given them by their appropriate zone of the earth or sky, so the social sciences and humanities are not realistic unless they admit, take their guidance from, the data given them by the history of human beings' performances, the record both past and present of what our kind of creature does. Paramount among such data is dying.

History and literature, two leading forms of humanistic inquiry, are shaped through and through by human mortality. Politics and economics contend every day with the fact that human beings need food, clothing, shelter, sex, medicine, and education for survival. The more profoundly a student of social science or the humanities studies these central issues, the more realistic and useful her or his results are likely to be. Creativity is not a matter of discovering new trivia. Creativity is a matter of shedding new light on old, central problems.

When I look for help with the old, central problem of terminal illness, I find little forthcoming from academe. Some faculty members of medical schools generate useful studies, but the university is not the powerhouse supplying new light on healing or suffering. Indeed, the suffering rampant in the university is the anxiety, the fear, the confusion of diseased spirits. The majority of the minds holding forth in our classrooms do not know what they believe, wonder whether belief itself is moral. The majority do not pray and are mute about love. Many love to teach, but less because they have a passion to share a truth, induct others into a beautiful vision, lay out a way to become holy than because they enjoy performing.

By and large, academic talk is brittle, polished but not strong. The mind generally honored is quick and verbal, not quiet and deep. To raise questions of value, religious import, or health in a profound sense is usually to be met with silence—either ignorance or embarrassment. To enter a general faculty meeting after a diagnosis of terminal cancer is to raise the level of anxiety and discomfort. In faculty meetings one is not dealing with people close to death and the peasant wisdoms that death teaches. One is dealing with people in flight from death, and from a lot of other realities.

I believe in education. I think that our primary responsibility as human beings is to gain sufficient understanding of ourselves and our world to live well. This makes me a philosopher, a lover of wisdom. It does not make me a possessor of wisdom. The love of wisdom is a process, a cast of mind and heart, a dynamism. In my case, it feels taken up by the Spirit of God, so as to become a venture in theology. But whether philosophical or theological, the wisdom that I find our human nature demanding is an embarrassment on most college campuses. It does not figure in the catalogues of courses, except marginally. It is lucky to make a fleeting, cumbersome, graceless appearance in the plans and speeches of college presidents and provosts, just before they get on to the heart of the academic venture, the budget.

Suppose that those in charge of higher education, and lower education for that matter, did not forget so systematically, so semi-deliberately, the centrality of death. Suppose that they did not repress the connatural truth that the main business of life, and so of realistic education, is to learn how to endure, negotiate with, maneuver through the radical mysteriousness of our condition. On such a supposition, meditation would become more significant than money and banking. Myths of creation and destiny would merit more prestige than the geometrics of cones. Sex, a primal lens of the radical mysteriousness of our human condition, would come in for a widespread, cross-disciplinary attention that might rescue it from the sniggers of the fraternity brothers. Healing could become a metaphor for a mending of bodies and minds that drew a new generation of young people into the Peace Corps, jobs corps, and the corps for teachers of poor people.

43. A Witness for Death

A sense of death provokes considerable anger at the folly, the culpable unreality, that I find in large institutions such as the church, medicine, and education. What is a stricken person to do? What witness is appropriate?

I do not feel comfortable playing John the Baptist, roaring out of the desert, eating locusts and denouncing all the pharisees. I am not Jesus, gentler but equally demanding. Maybe Elijah is a fitting model, here today and gone tomorrow, hiding out in the mountains, hearing God in a still small voice. Maybe my witness can be oracular, wry, forged by the irony that God needed cancer to get my attention.

I have come to think of the chemotherapy room as a demonstration chapel, where humble little liturgies teach me things to hand on to others. In the chemotherapy room, nobody knows the answer, so everyone is respectful. I cannot say what breast cancer or cancer of the colon implies, because I have not had them. I cannot even say what multiple myeloma necessitates, because each body is a new experiment. No pattern is ironclad.

Still, I can say that no guru who has not suffered a terminal illness warrants my full docility. No one who pontificates or dogmatizes about the meaning of serious illness really knows what he or she is talking about. This holds for the few patients who are mouthy, as well as for the few medical specialists who forget the difference between the knowing that is acquaintance and the knowing that is experience. Actually, the regular reticence of both patients and doctors is edifying. As things tend to work out, those who know do not speak. They listen.

A first mode of witnessing is listening. The beginning of wisdom, and also healing, is paying attention. The finest doctors and the wisest priests are the ones who are slow to proffer answers, interested first in what you have to say, where you are living, how you are doing, who God is making you into. The world is full of babblers. We all meet many who do not listen. We may not even speak to them because we know they are not interested. Rare are those who listen from the heart and offer you a fullness of silence. Precious are the few who extend a strong yet gentle compassion not because they can play a role well but because they are exceptionally human.

Terminal illness does not make anyone exceptionally human. It is only an occasion, not a cause. Pain has no necessary connection to wisdom. Without the grace of God, pain is more apt to brutalize us than sanctify us. Yet, wisdom does come through suffering, and Christ crucified exemplifies the Pauline power and wisdom of God. When talk of "wounded healers" is not simply voguish, passed from ear to lips without visiting the brain, it can name a hopeful truth. Our sufferings tend to purify us, if we let God use them. When we have no health in us, no comeliness to entice the outer world, we lose the power to impress others. We no longer keep people away because we are strong.

I used to worry about keeping people away because I was strong. Things had always gone easily for me, little was difficult. Even the abuses I suffered in childhood, from the church, and in academe seemed minor, nothing that far better people had not suffered less predictably. I took comfort in the fact that little children ventured close, were not frightened. Adults I did not know how not to judge, so I hid out and did my work, writing more books than was acceptable. A few people have interpreted my cancer as another mark of distinction, another barrier, but more people have thought they could approach closer now, seeing weakness, fatigue, brokenness.

The challenge will be to transmute these physical facts into a better interior listening. The chance that glimmers calls me to use the physical slowdown to curb impatience, mental quickness, and choler. I find dealing with other sick people easy, as I used to find dealing with the dying. I need now to see how all the people around me are sickly, even the physically robust. The shy are unsure of themselves, and so often are suffering. The cocksure are often stupid or shallow, another reason for compassion. Dealing patiently with the sick or slow is nothing special. Dealing patiently with the arrogant, the overbearing, the self-satisfied is a significant witness, still well beyond me most days. So I still have much to learn, many challenges to give my days meaning.

44. Preparing for Heaven

I believe that heaven is quite different from endless existence in the mode we now experience on earth. Seeing God, possessing God, loving God securely will make all the difference. Presently, however, there is no getting to heaven, no reaching the transformation that heaven connotes, except by passing through death.

Some mystics appear to enjoy a foretaste of heaven, through being taken into immediate union with God, but that cannot be the fullness of heaven or human consummation. Before death all human beings are less than fully transformed or penetrated by God's grace, divine life. It is not so much that, for full transformation, we have to leave the body as that we have to detach ourselves from its sin—its disorder, opacity, moral weakness. Death is not the end of the body, if resurrection is our destiny. But what death opens onto, how resurrection functions, none of us can know.

Sometimes I muse about these things, and they console me. The ability to move from my own particular pathos to the general pathos of all human beings seems a benefit of stepping back from critical illness, returning to the halfway house, the holding pattern, of remission. I suspect, ruefully, that much of my detachment may vanish, when my situation again becomes critical, but I hope, and pray, that some of it remains.

I am trying, in my meditations on death, to take deeply to heart, firmly into my soul, the serene hopes of longstanding Christian iconography. It is not easy to speak about heaven nowadays, for me not easy even to believe in heaven privately. But it is consoling to revisit what in prior ages was central to the mainstream culture. It brings me joy to remember Paul's assurances that we are not of all people the most to be pitied, because our faith in the resurrection is not vain.

I do not know whether my sense that death has become my neighbor, my intimate, is more than a wistful fancy. At times a visceral panic returns, unrebuffed by natural endorphins. None of us can guarantee the presence of the grace that lets us feel that all manner of thing will be well. But perhaps all of us can grow better at believing in the foundations of such blessedness.

Julian of Norwich, with whom I associate some of the most positive Christian conviction about the goodness of creation and the surety of our triumph over death, seems to be speaking from more than a transient mood. The deathbed experience that shaped her adult life, giving her endless food for reflection, occurred in the midst of terrible pain, yet it breathed into her spirit a boundless hope. Her God was so good, and so near, that evil lost its threat. The evil of death slunk away, because she had confronted it with the deathless being of God. The death of Christ revealed itself to be a supreme act of love, carried out completely for her benefit. Her sins mattered less than her faith. Salvation was there, fully accomplished. She had only to acknowledge it, fit herself to it. She had only to worship what God already was.

The other side of the silence I hear, when I pass beyond trouble to my depths, may be a symphony of what God already is. God, who always "was, is, and is to come," does not need explicit imagery to be the better of death, the conquerer of all negativity. I do not have to feel how God is more real than all my illusion and fear for God to be more real. I do well to bless the times, such as the present, when I can think these thoughts with fine feeling, letting images of hope bubble up from a peace beyond understanding—God can hold other times, the majority, when I am not so blessed.

All of us ought to ask God for the measures of feeling, illumination, and encouragement that we need. None of us is an angel, able to make do without sacraments. Perhaps we are wise to ask God to move us beyond feelings, beyond thoughts, even the most consoling, so that we can root ourselves in the being of God that the death and resurrection of Christ summon. But in the end God will give us the mixture of darkness and sacramentality that we need.

Indeed, we must believe that God gives the measures, the directives, that come through all our thoughts and moods. In fact, Christians can make their own the Buddhist conviction that every day is a good day, by thinking that all times come from God. Sickness never becomes good, if we stay within a physical horizon. Sickness only becomes good when we move to wider or deeper perspectives, where what sickness prompts, what we make of it, the illusions it destroys, the reforms it prompts come into focus.

I do not say this as easily as I might have said it several years ago, because the enormity of sickness rises up before me now, as it never could when I had not been seriously ill. Now I know at first hand that sometimes we can do no more than endure the pain, the disability, the dereliction that sickness thrusts upon us. Sometimes we cannot think clearly, and all we can feel is pain. God is nowhere that we can reach or imagine. Only the barest memory of reasons for thinking that God is everywhere may remain. All our faith in the goodness of God can seem vestigial.

Nonetheless, our dereliction need not defeat God. The return of calm, reliable reason makes this proposition indubitable. Nothing about us, whether good or bad, alive or infected with death, defeats God. God is God, regardless of what or how we are. God can be God for us, related to us knowingly and caringly, regardless of our feelings.

Jesus felt abandoned by God, forsaken, if we accept the plain words of the New Testament texts. God was not there, was missing, if the experience of Jesus, the awareness of Jesus, set the terms. Yet, the same texts go on to say that soon God acted in the depths of Jesus, so radically as to prompt images of a new creation, drawing

Jesus out of the jaws of death, making Jesus a new Jonah freed from leviathan. The God who was nowhere to be seen or felt made the abandonment of Jesus into the divine power and wisdom. "Take that to heart," I can say to my unbelieving, unfeeling spirit. "Think about Jesus the new Jonah."

45. Patient Endurance

I watch the behavior of other people seriously ill, especially those who have been at it longer than I, or whose situations are more dramatic. I note the modesty they tend to show, the many chances to pass judgment they forgo. Drawn more deeply into the divine mystery than the rest of us, they suffer little temptation to sell answers at bargain prices. The answers are obvious and will not be reduced. They will cost what the given illness exacts, no penny less or more. In a word, the answer is endurance, the patience in which, scripture says, we may possess our souls. In experience, patience becomes ineffable, wordless, a matter of being rather than saying.

The task set by terminal illness, the witness asked of our being, is to make it through the day. The day colors the task. Today I may have to endure pain, or depression, or torpor. The task, from God, is to bear it. Tomorrow I may have to ride herd on high spirits, false optimism, because for the moment I feel fine—tempted to forget my illness. Sufficient for each day is the task, the evil, thereof. Illness itself teaches us not to care about the morrow. The morrow may never come. If today we hear God's voice, we must not harden our hearts. God's voice can sound in ebb tide or in flood. Nothing limits God.

Talking with a friend who had just gone through surgery for thyroid cancer, I found myself asking whether she had been afraid. She said no, she had felt a great cushion of support. Listening hard, I could only say that that was wonderful, thinking that God had certainly been good. But then I heard myself dealing with the other side: "If that feeling of support goes, it doesn't mean anything."

I don't want that support to go. I don't think that desolation is more sanctifying than consolation. But I do think that both consolation and desolation are shaped intimately by our feelings, and that our feelings are imperfect indices of God. We have to use our feelings, because they are integral parts of ourselves. We can never become pure spirits, and should not want to be. But God is not limited to what we feel. God need not be missing because we cannot sense him. Our faith can go well beyond our feelings, just as our love can go well beyond our mind. Whether we live or die, feel fine or rotten, we belong to God. Whether we are good or bad, pious or sinful, we belong to God. Even when our hearts condemn us, God is greater. God is always greater—that is our surest ground.

People terminally ill have an exceptional opportunity to witness to others about the greatness of God. The opportunity comes like an engraved invitation, handed over on a silver platter. When my back broke from the action of the myeloma, I had little margin for detached thoughts or humor. For the first time in my life, crucifixion was not an abstraction. I found it ironic to ask

God why he had forsaken me. The hours before I could receive medication passed amazingly slowly. The ride to the emergency room in the ambulance took longer than I would have thought possible. At every bump, I wondered how atonement operates. Naked under a scratchy blanket, I remembered how I had come into the world. I could do nothing but hang on, try to endure, move into the pain, and so give it less space through which to gather momentum and belt me. In none of this was there was anything romantic or heroic. I was glad I was alone in the back of the ambulance, that no one else had to witness my writhing.

Ideally we should handle terminal illness or other heavy trouble with prayer as Jesus has counseled us. The best course is probably to close the door and address our heavenly Father in secret. Yes, we have to move through the world. We are bound to bear a persona for public consumption, but the less this is a mask, a matter of conscious design, the better for all involved. We are what we are, for better or worse, richer or poorer. We owe others nothing but what we are, no gimmicks or special performances. Yes, if being aware of others makes us braver, we should be aware gladly. In the hospital, surrounded by largely female caregivers, I was amused to find sexual roles continuing. Flat on my back, gray and unshaven, I still wanted to play the handsome marine. Even more, though, I wanted to make it through the day. If playing the marine, keeping a stiff upper lip, made making it through the day easier, fine and dandy. In my broken bones, though, I knew that if crying were more useful, I was a fool not to cry.

The people who helped me think best about what was wise endurance and what foolish were the terminally ill people I had known. Two friends, in particular, had shared with me their experience of terminal cancer, and both had been real men. I remembered their honesty, their desire to evade nothing. I remembered their faith: solid but understated. So I made myself slow to give out pious phrases, determined to register life as it was actually occurring. Good days were to be called good. Bad days were not to be fudged. The surprising thing was that good days outnumbered bad, even when I was in miserable shape. Morphine or the grace of God or the prayers of my stricken wife kept me from breaking or crashing. Any good witness from this, though, came in the fact, not in a smiley exegesis.

You, God, are too real for our words. Only our beings approach you. We know you through the ways you deal with us, hobbling along week after week. A cloud by day, a pillar of fire at night, you come and go as you choose. This is how we find you, so this should be our witness. You are not God as we think of you. You are God as you show yourself to be.

46. From Shock to Acceptance

Nearly two years after receiving my diagnosis of multiple myeloma, I no longer find it shocking. Occasionally, late at night or in the dark before dawn, I find it unreal. On the many days when I feel normal, except for a sore back and leg, I wonder whether my cancer is not some sort of a dream.

The assault of the first weeks has subsided. The earthquake continues to summon vivid memories, and to have strong consequences, but the ground no longer trembles.

For the moment, then, I may occupy a privileged microzone, high enough above normal, unthreatened existence to offer a long view, yet low enough not to make me dizzy. If the summer when my cancer first occurred brought the worst physical pain of my life, the following summer brought the best mental health I have ever experienced.

Self-deception is always possible, but I think I am seeing clearly. What I see commits me to the nearly tautological position that what will be will be, and I find this commitment wise religiously. When I pray for my friends and benefactors, above all those who have prayed for me and Denise in this time of suffering, I ask God to give them abandonment to what will be. May they agree, down to the fine point of their souls, that God numbers their days for their benefit. May not a breeze waft, not a drop of rain fall, except, in their eyes, as an expression of God's love for them. All God's ways are ways of love. The alternative is unthinkable: a God less admirable than our own human hearts.

Acceptance need not be passive. I am not advocating the quietism that orthodox Christians have always condemned. I am not saying that we human beings have no work to do, no part to play in our own living and dying well. I do not forget that we are to love our neighbors as we love ourselves, and that if we do not love the brother or sister whom we can see, our claims to love the God whom we cannot see are dubious.

Indeed, I like the emphasis that liberation theology places on praxis. I think that the American pragmatists were quite biblical when they made deeds the criterion of claims, and not vice versa. After all, bad people hate the light *because* their deeds are evil. We can know whether people are bad, or good, by their fruits—the deeds they do, the love they lay on the line.

I have been testing my faith, trying to discern my love, by the way I have been living—holding up, working and loving, day by day. I have downgraded the importance of my feelings, including my aches and pains. Instead I have concentrated on my degree of abandonment to divine providence. Recalling de Caussade, Brother Lawrence, Saint Thérèse, and the parables of Jesus, I have tried to make myself indifferent to what happens. According to Paul, whether I live or die, I am the Lord's. According to Jesus, my heavenly Father, blessed Mother, knows all that I need.

I see no sane alternative to this acceptance, this abandonment to divine providence. It is not an intellectual position that I elect so much as a necessity for spiritual survival. To make it through the day, I need to believe that God has a purpose for all our doings, especially all our sufferings. Village atheism puts me off, and I find the brass of those who refuse to think about these things ugly and tarnished.

T. S. Eliot saw that we undergo much more than we accomplish. Properly understood, acceptance, passivity, is how the Christian Taoist prospers. The Way, the will of God, moves the ten thousand things, regardless of our feelings. Whether we agree or disagree, the sun shines, the rain falls, on just and unjust alike. The Spirit breathes where it will, not waiting on our compliance. The trick of the spiritual life, our maturation in realism, is to sail by the Spirit's breathing.

To the end of our days, at both the peaks and the valleys of our creativity, we remain the clay pots, not the potter. The mystery always precedes us, supports us, draws us forward. The God who was, is, and will be measures all our time but is personally unmeasured. If this God spells out our fate with the word "cancer," we are wise to think our illness previewed, predestined, from time out of mind. The "double predestination" of the Calvinists can be brilliant, but I find de Caussade's blank check more telling.

None of us stands righteous before God, and no signs of election are certain. God can raise up children of

Abraham, elect, from inert stones. I cannot know the ultimate state of my soul, and you cannot know the ultimate state of yours. All human beings have sinned and fallen short of God's glory. The salvation of any one of us is a work of grace.

For all of us, then, acceptance is an acceptance of grace. We would not even know that we could be saved, were it not for the biblical witness that culminates in Jesus. Left to ourselves, we could only hope to imitate Socrates or the Buddha, and become people of good conscience, people who would follow the light if they saw it, would rejoice to see the morning star.

47. The Morning Star

When you are terminally ill, the morning star is precious. Seeing it, you realize that you have made it through another night, that the darkness has not yet conquered you. Often I think of Saint John of the Cross, who wrote so well of spiritual darkness. In his view, the less sensible our faith, the better our commitment to God.

If the Christian ideal is to love God for God's own sake, rather than for the gifts, material or spiritual, that God might bestow on us, then darkness can be better than sunshine, quiet better than drama. How things go in our spirit is determined by God's Spirit. We are most believing when we let God parcel out our bread, our wine, day by day.

Today I have no reason to think that my multiple myeloma has resurged. Tomorrow I may have reason. Today I thank God for prolonging my remission. Tomorrow I may have to thank God for ending it. Presently, I am far better at thanking God for health than thanking God for illness. But the logic of abandonment, the line that John of the Cross draws in the sand, leads to the conclusion that every day can be a good day. In fact, sickness can be no less a gift than health, Ignatius of Loyola said. The principle and foundation of the Christian spiritual life is that our only reason-to-be is to serve and praise God. If our living serves and praises God, so be it. If our dying serves and praises God, so be it. It is up to God to determine whether we live or die. It is up to us to say, mean, embrace "so be it."

God offers intimacy with the divine persons, the trinitarian community, through the ordinary events of our daily lives. Karl Rahner's "supernatural existential" hypothesizes that there is no purely natural situation, no place material or spiritual where the trinitarian community does not constitute the deepest reality. Inasmuch as we live in good conscience, trying to discern the signs of the times and respond faithfully, we say yes to the offer that God is making.

Accepting our circumstances, our selves, our history, we open our hearts to God's self-gift. We did not make the world, and the portions of the world that we can change are minor. Certainly, we must do what we can to preserve nature and make human environments in which people can thrive. But what we can do is limited. The first job of any healthy culture is to make people realistic. People who deny the universality of death, who live as though death could not come like a thief on this very night, are not realistic. Similarly, people who think that anything human can fulfill them are not realistic. They are ignoring both the testimony of the sages and the testimony of their own experience.

Acceptance, though, is more than enduring or coming to love the divine darkness. It has its glorious aspects, and I would be remiss not to mention them. Human experience embraces more than death and limitation. There is beauty in the skies, the fields, the eyes of other people. There is love to make the soul sing, prayer to ravish the spirit.

Creative work is a gift of God, reknitting the raveled sleeve of care better than sleep. The endurance of injustice, unowed suffering, bears witness to the holiness of God, whether or not the witness realizes it. The birth of new children is a marvel, a reason to shout out thanks to God. The death of elderly people in peace is a reason to pray thanks quietly. Music and art, science and serving the poor—the other reasons are numerous.

If there is a daunting mystery of iniquity, there is at least a balancing mystery of goodness. If nothingness can dog all our days, paint over everything in creation, there is yet the marvelous question of why there should be something, being rather than nothingness.

Now and then people love their enemies, do good to those who persecute them. Now and then saints make the law of the cross persuasive: Love is stronger than death, stronger than evil. Love can redeeem our lives from the pit. After Jesus, we need not speak of Sheol. In his wake, his light, his footsteps, we can speak of heaven: hymns to the Lamb who was slain. He is worthy, even though we are not. He can receive all power and glory and honor and might, because he is the first-born from the dead and Lord of all. God from God, Light from Light, he is as endless as the Father. When we accept his lordship, we receive their Spirit, who makes our deepest, groaning prayer: "Abba." Into those hands we may commend our spirit.

48. *Prayer and the Absolute Future*

We commend our spirits, and those of all whom we love, for whom we are responsible, at prayer. We interact with God, speaking and listening, through prayer. Prayer is this interaction, this commending. Prayer is to the human spirit what food and drink are to the body.

Prayer is not so much thought as love. It can feel lovely, speak beautifully, double itself by singing, but it need not. Prayer can be our bare selves, down and out, barely hanging on. It can come out of the depths: *De profundis clamavi ad te.* Did you hear me? Did my cry at least echo in heaven? Speak, Lord, that your servant may hear you. Grant me your small still voice.

The variations on prayer and permutations on crying are endless. If we go to the highest heavens, the angels of God ferry our joy. If we fall to the lowest abysses, the nadir of sin, the lamb of God remains slain for our sake, the source of blood to wash us whiter than snow.

Prayer is our passion, the suffering of our spirit under heaven. It is our action, what we do from the heart to say yes to God. The saints in heaven pray constantly, praising God every hour. The angels cry "holy, holy, holy": *trisagion.* Every godward movement is prayerful. Need and hope, thanks and petition—all motion, every relation, is oration, *oraison.*

When I think of the absolute future, the end of the tunnel toward which my cancer is hurtling me, I sometimes realize that the future is now. The eschaton, the end-time, is this present, acceptable hour. That is the great message of Johannine spirituality, and the reason it is the most sacramental. Here, now, in this space, this time, the absolute future can be present. When the eternal Word took flesh, salvation became permanent. Once, and for all, what human beings, indeed all creatures, postulate—demand from the core of their beings—made itself available, and it promised never to leave.

The Lord has sworn and will not repent. The Creator has pitched a tent in creation. Certainly, creation still groans as though in labor, waiting for the fullness of its redemption. Obviously, we have here no lasting city, no new Jerusalem come down from heaven like a bride bedecked for her husband, blessed be He. But we have here the substance of those things, the prolepsis, the promise. We have the symbols bubbling up from the substance, the down-payment, the *arrabon*. In a word, we have the Spirit, the Paraclete. We have a heavenly helper, cheerleader, advocate, maker of prayer.

God is the absolute future, and Christian faith insists that God is nigh. The sacraments that actualize formally the sacramentality following on the Incarnation never fail to anoint time making it holy. I have received all seven sacraments (once only an anomalous possibility). I have been baptized, confirmed, forgiven, ordained, married, anointed, and fed with the bread of angels. Every time, grace has become tangible, prayer has brought the absolute future into a given place, a given time, creating a holy moment. Whether I was distracted or recollected, appreciative or sullen, the moment occurred, the miracle happened. That is the essence of what we mean by the church: the place where sacrament and word happen most formally.

The church is the eschatological, complete and unfailing, community of salvation, expressing itself fully trustworthily through Word and Sacrament. This is the reason that we who constitute the church are the people of God, why we stand out in the world, like a city raised high on the mountain.

I have to flee the world to find the church. I have to flee the worldly, predominant parts of my own consciousness. I have to read books that are holy, brimming with faith. I do not find the church in *The New York Times*. Other Christians, blessed with faith stronger than mine, can find the church, the grace of God, signs of salvation everywhere. On my own, I seldom can. My spirit is too impressionable, too malleable. My spirit is a whore, going wherever the payoff glistens. So, I have to discipline my spirit, insist that it set aside time for reading good books, time for thinking about holy things, time for praying, ideally wordlessly, worldlessly, out of the depths. Even with discipline, I forget about the absolute future more than I remember it. I fear the medical future more than I wait for it patiently as the disposition of God.

49. Jesus the Savior

Lately a discussion, perhaps even a controversy, has blazed (not really raged) about whether Jesus, the Christ, is the absolute savior. In light of the good effects of the Buddha, Muhammad, and other holy worthies, should we Christians not, in ecumenical honesty, modesty, and generosity, reduce the absoluteness of our claims for the salvation effected by, available in, Jesus? Should we not stop confessing, claiming, that forgiveness from God, life forever with God, comes through no other name? Certainly, God remains the absolute, of the past and present as well as the future. But how can Jesus, fully human like ourselves, be the unique bringer of salvation from God, the solely adequate enfleshment, the only fully efficacious sacrament?

Simply. We need only recite the traditional creeds, say yes to the longstanding offer, and Jesus the Christ, the Word become flesh, becomes Jesus-for-us, the alpha and omega for anyone. If Jesus is divine, then communion with Jesus, union with him in love, makes us divine by participation. If no other human being is divine as Jesus is, as the enfleshment of the Word of God, then the communion we can have with any other human being, what we can become through loving participation, is not divinity of the same sort, to the same degree, with the same implications for salvation (rescue from sin, establishment in wholeness), that communion with Jesus, through faith and hope and love inspired by the Spirit of Jesus, entails.

Despite the endless proliferation of possible distinctions, qualifications, difficulties, or amendments, I find the heart of the controversy simple. If I accept the high Christology, the full confession of the divinity of Jesus the Christ, that the New Testament legitimates and the conciliar creeds bring to unmistakable clarity, there is only one Word incarnate, one absolute savior. Only once did the Word spoken eternally in the bosom of the Father take flesh of a sister of ours and so fix eternity to a specific personal history, make one lifetime the story of God.

I think it is important to get all the clarity one can on this matter. People are not saved by the words they create, the ideas they have, the orthodoxy they do or do not seem to manifest. People are saved by the love in their hearts, the yes they say in their depths to the joys and sufferings God gives them.

One can confess Jesus to be the absolute savior and still find salvation flourishing among people who have never heard of Jesus. Salvation can also be found among people (such as Muslims or Jews) whose faith explicitly denies the divinity of Jesus. I also think that anyone, healthy or sickly, who opens himself or herself to the absolute mystery of God is a Christian at least anonymously, unknowingly. I think this latter thought because I find the life of Jesus the Christ to be the paradigm for human authenticity, human success, wherever found, however expressed in terms of culture and lifestyle.

Jesus discloses the absolute future to be a personal holiness, goodness, loveliness that we can trust unreservedly. Despite rejection, abuse, terrible suffering, Jesus continued to trust his heavenly Father. The implications of what Jesus was (such a truster, such a believer) and how Jesus lived (with blazing honesty and love), apply always and everywhere as a revelation applicable universally. Nowhere else do I see enfleshed, incarnated, sacramentalized so clearly or deeply the faith, hope, and love that make the future absolutely good, trustworthy, for-us. Though I find goodness and wisdom in many other places, those other places, those other personal revelations, are less adequate expressions, incarnations, translations of the goodness of God, the graciousness of the absolute future, than what I find in Jesus. So I make Jesus the explicator of the salvation available in those other places, and I make Jesus the explicand at their heart or foundation. Jesus is both what I must explain, if I am to clarify the history or enfleshment of what Muslim or Buddhist holiness entails, and how I am to explain it.

Naturally, this depends on my Christian faith, my prior commitment to Jesus because of the adequacy and the beauty that I find in him. But I cannot give up this dependency, this Christianness of my faith, when I move into ecumenical dialogue, any more than I can give it up when I go into the hospital chapel and gaze at the crucifix. Ecumenical dialogue cannot become more basic than my faith, nor can my cancer.

My faith, the Christ at the center of everything that I believe, that makes me me, is the determinant of my interpretational horizon and can never be the determined. It is the beginning, the end, the operator, not the secondary, the penultimate, the operated upon. Certainly, I can imagine giving up this determinative faith, this absolutely saving Christ, but what I imagine then is no longer Christian. It no longer embodies the high, strong, absolute sense that "Christian" carried for the saints who died for Jesus, that I would like it to carry for me still, apart from this hypothetical, imaginary change that I have just described.

You may think that my need of an absolute savior, my fear of death, or something else drives me to absolutize Jesus and make Christian tradition similarly absolutizing. You may be right. I don't know, for sure, and neither do you, neither can you. Something parallel drives you to deabsolutize Jesus, some parallel need works in you, if you are a reformer bent on denying the uniqueness of Jesus, bent on finding in some other name a salvation you think just as good.

The psychological game of sniffing for motives can be extended to any of us, applies as much on one side of the fence as the other. You may think that you are more mature, or generous ecumenically, for deabsolutizing Jesus. You may be right, but you cannot know for certain, any more than I can. We both have to wait for a final judgment, an arbitration that we can only reach through death. You have grounds for anticipating this calmly, but so do I. We both have reasons for tact and tolerance, reasons as near as our equal ignorance.

This is a debate, a controversy, that I leave outside the chapel. When I pray my way toward the absolute future, I don't argue about the absoluteness of Christ. At my best moments, I focus on the cross of Christ simply, without words or arguments, trying only to let it be my summary statement, what I move toward God in front of me, as my defense. It is the exegesis of my desire, the sign of the love that I wish I had, that I would like to show. The more Christian my prayer, the less I am present, the more Jesus predominates. He must increase. We must decrease. That is the law of Christian faith, codified long ago by John the Baptizer.

The Jesus who predominates in orthodox, admirable Christian faith is alive, the first-born from the dead and lord of all. He is the blazing figure of the Book of Revelation, with the voice of many waters. He is the morning star, and the champion who rides out from heaven. He has slain death, crushed the prior strong man and retaken the house made of dawn. He is more than any poetry, least of all mine. So I find myself saying, "Maranatha." I murmur, in good times and in bad, "Come God, my death."

Of Related Interest...

The Pummeled Heart
Finding Peace Through Pain
Antoinette Bosco

A sensitive, faith-filled and heart-rending journey through one woman's life, showing how the difficulties encountered along the way can become the basis for true growth.

ISBN: 0-89622-584-4, 140 pp, $7.95

Caring for Yourself When Caring for Others
Margot Hover

Hover offers ways for caregivers to nourish themselves, and thereby revitalize their efforts. This book is for all caregivers, from parents with young children to medical professionals.

ISBN: 0-89622-533-x, 80 pp, $7.95

Body, Mind & Spirit
To Harmony through Meditation
Louis Hughes

The author offers simple exercises conducive to prayer that relax the body and mind while freeing the spirit.

ISBN: 0-89622-484-8, 128 pp, $7.95

Available at religious bookstores or from

TWENTY-THIRD PUBLICATIONS
P.O. Box 180 • Mystic, CT 06355

1-800-321-0411